Strong Women, Strong Hearts

MIRIAM E. NELSON, PH.D., AND

ALICE H. LICHTENSTEIN, D.SC.

with

LAWRENCE LINDNER, M.A.

*Friedman School of Nutrition Science
and Policy, Tufts University*

◆

G. P. PUTNAM'S SONS

New York

Strong Women,
Strong Hearts

◆

PROVEN STRATEGIES TO

PREVENT AND REDUCE

HEART DISEASE

NOW

G. P. PUTNAM'S SONS
Publishers Since 1838
Published by the Penguin Group
Penguin Group (USA) Inc., 375 Hudson Street, New York, New York 10014, USA • Penguin
Group (Canada), 10 Alcorn Avenue, Toronto, Ontario M4V 3B2, Canada (a division of Pearson Penguin
Canada Inc.) • Penguin Books Ltd, 80 Strand, London WC2R 0RL, England • Penguin Ireland,
25 St Stephen's Green, Dublin 2, Ireland (a division of Penguin Books Ltd) • Penguin Group
(Australia), 250 Camberwell Road, Camberwell, Victoria 3124, Australia (a division of Pearson Australia
Group Pty Ltd) • Penguin Books India Pvt Ltd, 11 Community Centre, Panchsheel Park,
New Delhi–110 017, India • Penguin Group (NZ), cnr Airborne and Rosedale Roads, Albany,
Auckland 1310, New Zealand (a division of Pearson New Zealand Ltd) • Penguin Books (South Africa)
(Pty) Ltd, 24 Sturdee Avenue, Rosebank, Johannesburg 2196, South Africa
Penguin Books Ltd, Registered Offices: 80 Strand, London WC2R 0RL, England

Library of Congress Cataloging-in-Publication Data

Nelson, Miriam E.
Strong women, strong hearts: proven strategies to prevent and reduce heart
disease now / by Miriam E. Nelson and Alice H. Lichtenstein with Lawrence Lindner.
p.   cm.
Includes bibliographical references and index.
ISBN 0-399-15287-3
1. Heart diseases in women—Popular works.   2. Heart diseases in women—prevention.
I. Lichtenstein, Alice H.   II. Lindner, Lawrence.   III. Title.
RC682.N445   2005   2004058734
616.1'205'082—dc22

Printed in the United States of America
1   3   5   7   9   10   8   6   4   2

This book is printed on acid-free paper. ∞

PAR-Q questionnaire on pages 104–105 reprinted with permission of Canada Society for Exercise Physiology.
    Exercise intensity scales on pages 114 and 118 used with permission from Miriam E. Nelson, Ph.D., with
Sarah Wernick, Ph.D., *Strong Women Stay Young* (New York: Bantam Books, 2000).
    Select recipes on pages 94–96 used with permission from Miriam E. Nelson, Ph.D., with Judy Knipe, *Strong
Women Eat Well* (G. P. Putnam's Sons, 2001).
    Illustrations by Wendy Wray/Vicki Morgan Associates, NYC.

For our daughters

An Important Caution

◆

The advice given in *Strong Women, Strong Hearts* is based on extensive scientific research. This book contains instructions and safety precautions. It is essential that you read them carefully. Some exercises are inappropriate for individuals with heart disease or other medical conditions.

This book is not intended to replace the services of a health care provider who knows you personally. An essential element of taking responsibility for your health is having regular checkups and working in partnership with medical professionals.

If you are under treatment for heart disease or any other medical condition—or if you suspect you might need such care—you must discuss this program with your doctor before you begin.

Contents

◆

Preface

◆

Going on two years ago, I was walking into our research center at Tufts one day when a colleague, Dr. Alice Lichtenstein, stopped me in the hallway. I had written books about osteoporosis, arthritis, weight control, and other conditions, she said, but why hadn't I yet written *Strong Women, Strong Hearts*? After all, she argued, there is perhaps no more important impact that exercise and good nutrition have on health than to reduce the risk of heart disease. On top of that, Alice said, more women die of heart disease each year than men, but most women aren't aware of that. They need to hear about it, and they need to learn what to do to avoid it.

She was right, of course. But I looked at her and responded, "Alice, that's *your* book to write." Alice is one of the world's finest scientists in the field of nutrition and heart disease; she heads the Cardiovascular Nutrition Laboratory at Tufts and currently chairs the Nutrition Committee of the American Heart Association.

"We need to talk," she said. "Without you and your expertise in physical activity, we don't have the crucial exercise component."

A week later, I met with Alice to discuss collaborating on this book. And soon after that, we were putting together *Strong Women, Strong Hearts* with our collaborator, Larry Lindner, who brought his writing talent to bear on the project.

Preparing this book with Alice has been an incredibly rich experience, one that you might say was twenty years in the making. I remember very well when, as a graduate student in 1984, I listened enthralled on those days she appeared as a new-graduate guest lecturer in my nutritional biochemistry class. I remember being in awe of her command of the science, her ability to explain the intricacies of dietary fats and carbohydrates. I was fascinated by her explanations of what happens to food once it is absorbed; how it gets metabolized and increases or decreases the risk for chronic disease.

I am learning from Alice still. There was much I learned, in fact, during the writing of this book (and, she insisted I include here, much she learned from me).

We both hope that you learn, too, as you read—and are inspired to take steps to protect yourself. Premature death and disability from heart disease can be largely eliminated if women make the choice to eat better and exercise more.

From both Alice and me, here's to strong women—with very strong hearts.

Miriam Nelson

PART 1

Women and Heart Disease— Where Are We Now?

CHAPTER 1

A Call to Action

◆

I was first diagnosed with borderline high blood pressure in my twenties, when I was pregnant. I still had high blood pressure after I gave birth, but I was told only that I had to go on a strict diet even though I wasn't really overweight. I went like that for years, with my blood pressure getting higher and higher throughout my thirties. Not until I was in my forties and my blood pressure skyrocketed to 200 over 100 was I given medication to lower it.

—LINDA

I woke up one morning with severe chest pain, severe upper back pain, nauseated, short of breath—an overall horrible feeling. It got worse and worse throughout the day. Finally, I went to the emergency room. The doctor said, "It's probably just a muscle. . . . I'm going to give you a muscle relaxant and send you home." But as much as I was rationalizing ("Did I play racquetball too hard? Could this be food poisoning?"), I had this sense of doom. I didn't want to leave until I had had further testing. "I want an EKG," I said. "I want a blood test." Reluctantly, they agreed. When they first attached me to the EKG machine, the nurse thought she had hooked me up wrong. She called in another nurse. Then they got the doctor. It took twenty minutes for them to finally believe I was having a heart attack.

—CINDY

I had to wait thirty minutes in the emergency room. They thought I had indigestion and sent me home with very strong pain medication. I was back in the emergency room late that night. They finally did an EKG— and immediately air-lifted me to a larger hospital for emergency heart surgery. I stopped breathing on the table.

—DeLinda

HEART DISEASE KILLS MORE WOMEN THAN MEN

Unfortunately, what happened to these women is not unique. Heart disease is considered a man's problem, but every year since 1984, it has killed more women than men in the United States. A woman dies from heart disease about once every minute, for an annual total of about half a million deaths.

There are also lots of women *living* with heart disease—some eight million.

It has clearly reached a crisis point, one that reflects an unfortunate irony. So much has been made of women's hearts as symbols—of love, purity of emotion, the center of a home. But the female heart can become diseased, and the very realness of the heart as giver of life is ignored.

Even if a woman *is* properly diagnosed, she is often not properly tended to:

- Whereas 25 percent of men die within one year of a first heart attack, the number surges to 38 percent for women.
- Eighteen percent of male heart attack survivors experience a second heart attack within six years, compared with 35 percent of women heart attack sufferers—almost twice the proportion.
- Women are almost two times as likely as men to die after bypass surgery, and half as likely to get an angioplasty to open a narrowed blood vessel.

Unfortunately, stubborn myths about women and heart disease stand in the way of effective treatment.

Myth: When it comes to women, it's more important to focus on breast cancer than heart disease.

Fact: Heart disease is the leading killer of women in the United States, taking many times more lives than breast cancer. Breast cancer is a devastating disease, but you can't deny the numbers. Heart disease kills 499,000 women each year (compared with 432,000 men). Breast cancer kills 40,000 women each year.

Myth: It's men who need to be the focus of lifestyle changes for preventing heart disease.

Fact: Women need to protect themselves by living heart-healthfully, too—but often don't. In a University of Nebraska Medical Center study that looked at almost 200 couples in which the man had had a heart attack or by-pass surgery, it was found that in one in three households, *both* husbands and wives were overweight, and they ate similar amounts of fat and salt. There were also similarities in their exercise levels as well as in their smoking histories. Indeed, women were twice as likely as their husbands to continue smoking eight weeks after their spouse's heart attack or heart surgery. *Many of the women did not even know their own blood cholesterol levels,* which, as we will explain, is an essential piece of knowledge for each of us.

Myth: A low-fat diet is the best thing for your heart.

Fact: The advice from the scientific community is no longer to keep dietary fat as low as possible. In fact, for some people, very low-fat diets can actually contribute to heart disease. The goal now is to keep only certain types of fat as low as possible. The limit for fats in general has been liberalized. Even up to 35 percent of calories from fat is now considered acceptable (as long as it doesn't contribute to weight gain).

Myth: If you've been diagnosed with heart disease, you should not exercise.

Fact: If you've been diagnosed with heart disease, it is more important than ever to exercise. Gone are the weeks of bed rest for heart attack patients. Most are now encouraged to start moving their bodies again as soon as possible, even before they leave the hospital. Those with heart-related risk factors, such as high cholesterol, should be challenging their hearts to work harder with exercise, too.

Myth: Heart disease is an inevitable consequence of aging.

Fact: No, it's not. Yes, growing older puts you at higher heart disease risk. But risk is just that: risk. It's not a foregone conclusion, even for those with a family history of heart disease. There's much you can do in your everyday life to thwart "fate."

THE FEMALE HEART STEPS INTO THE SPOTLIGHT

The tide is shifting. As recently as 1958, paying attention to women's heart health was such an anomaly that heart disease researchers reporting on one of their studies noted it was "the first time that any members of the 'weaker sex' had participated in this work." Today, that patronizing observation has been replaced with a policy handed down from the federal government that half of all subjects in heart disease studies *must* be women in order for research funding to continue.

And the momentum is building. Only last year, both the American Heart Association (AHA) and the National Heart, Lung, and Blood Institute began campaigns to put women's heart disease risk front and center. The AHA's campaign, a "national call for women to take charge of their heart health and live stronger, longer lives," is called Go Red for Women. The National Heart, Lung, and Blood Institute's program is known as "The Heart Truth: A National Awareness Campaign on Women and Heart Disease." The AHA is the largest health advocacy organization focused on heart disease and stroke, and the National Heart, Lung, and Blood Institute is *the* major government agency focused on cardiovascular disease. These changes represent an enormous step forward.

The push to put the spotlight on women and heart disease comes not a moment too soon. It's especially pressing in light of all the recent negative findings on the effects of hormone replacement therapy (HRT). For years, women were told that HRT would protect them from heart disease, and millions took it believing they were not only relieving menopausal symptoms and helping their bones but also taking care of their cardiovascular systems. Now, rigorously conducted research has concluded that there is a slight but significant increase in the risk for heart attacks with HRT—even within the first year of use.

With the HRT avenue of heart protection closed off, more than ever women need straightforward guidelines about how to take action to avoid their biggest killer—and how to take care of themselves should heart disease strike.

The good news: Those guidelines are just coming together. The research on what women can do to protect themselves has reached the critical point at which it can be "translated" for use, which is why we've written this book *now*.

NO MATTER WHERE YOU'RE STARTING FROM . . .

While you cannot change your genes or your age, there's much you *can* do to keep heart disease at bay, or lessen its severity should it ever occur. That's true no matter what your starting fitness level, your current dietary habits, or whether you're pre- or postmenopausal. Even if you've already been diagnosed with heart disease, you can dramatically reduce your risk that it will get worse. It's *never* too late to make a difference. You can start today with strategies that are entirely in your own control.

Strong Women, Strong Hearts lays it all out in terms you can understand—a complete program that guides you through, step by step. There's nutrition, physical activity, weight control, relaxation and de-stressing techniques, and much more. For instance, one of the most important components of living a heart-healthy lifestyle is diet, which is why we devote an entire chapter to that topic. The right eating pattern for heart health can reduce the risk for a future heart attack or stroke dramatically, yet it is one aspect of the heart protection issue that has become especially confusing. Is it low-fat and high-carbohydrate? High-protein and low-carbohydrate? What about soy—and oatmeal? Do they really lower cholesterol? Are red meat and eggs "bad"? How much fish is right, especially given all the reports of contaminants in seafood?

To help you pull it all together, we distill the best research on the subject (some from our very own research groups and colleagues' laboratories) to offer a mix-and-match menu plan that allows you to choose the foods *you* prefer so that you'll stick with it. It works no matter what your eating style. There's no food *prescription*. While what you choose to eat can work as powerfully as medicine to keep down your heart disease risk, it should be *enjoyed*, not swallowed as a bitter pill.

Along with sound, flexible nutrition guidelines, we show you the latest in exercise to keep your heart primed as well as possible. It's not just aerobic exercises that count—walking, running, swimming, biking, and the like. There's now convincing research that strength training is also very important for the conditioning of the entire cardiovascular system.

Even if you've never walked a mile or lifted a dumbbell in your life (an all-too-likely scenario since 76 percent of women are sedentary), you'll be able to acclimate yourself to this plan, outlined in the chapter on exercise. We give step-by-step instructions so that you can work up to a desirable fitness level *gradually*. You'll never be at a loss for what to do, how to measure your progress, or how fast to go.

Those women who need to lose weight to lower their heart disease risk—or keep their weight from creeping up—will also get step-by-step instructions. We outline *the* ten strategies any woman should follow to lose weight healthfully. You'll be amazed, even though you have to keep at it, at how much flexibility there is to a healthful weight-management plan *that works*.

While some chapters get at your heart through your eating habits and physical activity patterns, chapter 8 gets at your heart through your *soul*. Research has convincingly shown that your outlook in life—how angry you tend to get, how you channel that anger, how you connect with others, whether you are spiritually connected, and so on—has a lot to do with the state of your heart. To that end, we offer strategies you can follow to get in touch with both yourself and those around you. That connectedness, in turn, will protect your heart from insidious damage it can sustain from the stresses of day-to-day life.

There's also the manner in which you look out for yourself. Or do you? A lot of women tend to accommodate everyone else before themselves—at the expense of not only their own happiness but also their health. Women end up *dying* because they're so busy taking care of others that they don't stop to take care of themselves. The tendency not to challenge the status quo—leaving the doctor's office without answers to their questions, leaving the hospital without *really* having been taken care of, sacrificing their own needs in order not to "make waves"—undercuts their ability to protect their hearts in very serious ways. In chapter 11, through one woman's life-and-death struggle to get her heart tended to, we advise you on how to *advocate* for yourself so that you get the help you need.

There is also a separate chapter on medications you might be prescribed to lower blood cholesterol or blood pressure and a chapter on procedures you may undergo to either help diagnose a heart problem or fix one—angiograms, bypasses, heart valve replacements, and the like. We feel it is very important to have a handle on what you're going through, or about to go through. That will allow you to ask the right questions as you get the care you need and in no small way relieve anxiety about medical therapies that you might otherwise be unfamiliar with. When anxiety is relieved, you will have more mental energy left to take the best possible care of yourself.

But long before you read through those chapters, you'll get a basic understanding of how a heart—how a *woman's* heart—works, in chapter 2. The research underpinnings of all the lifestyle advice we have culled together will be explained early on, too, so you'll know *why* we're suggesting what we suggest.

You'll also be asked to answer several questions about yourself so you can ascertain your level of heart disease risk in the first place. Do you know your blood cholesterol level? Your level of physical fitness? Your blood pressure?

If not, you're not alone. Despite the advances, as an exercise physiologist (Miriam Nelson) and a heart disease researcher (Alice Lichtenstein), we are all too aware that many women's risk for cardiovascular illness is higher than they may realize. Indeed, it has meaning for us in a personal way, as it does for you. As women in middle age, we never want to be counted among the grim statistics ourselves. Nor do we want our daughters to be as they make their way through adolescence toward adulthood. The same sentiment goes for our older friends and relatives. We don't think *any* woman should be a heart disease target—which is why we've pulled together the latest research on women and heart disease and written this book.

We feel it's our *responsibility* to share the accumulated knowledge about how to stave off cardiovascular illness in women, just as it is now *your* responsibility to give voice to the issue and share your newfound knowledge with others. The more women speak up—and make full use of the tools available—the greater the strides we can make.

It's time to put an end to the myth that heart disease wears only a shirt and tie, that women are immune from cardiovascular problems, that women don't need to take just as much care of their hearts as men do of theirs. By reading this book and following its guidelines, you're upending that myth and taking charge of your heart, in more ways than one.

What Makes a Woman's Heart Unique?

◆

I told my internist I had been having heartburn for three weeks and that my teeth ached. It was really more jaw pain, as if I were getting an electric shock in my jaw. She diagnosed gastric reflux and prescribed heartburn medicine. About thirty-six hours later, I had a major heart attack. I was 40.

—JUDY

When it comes to affairs of the heart, women definitely differ from men, whose heart disease often hits like a Mack truck rather than in the form of the more subtle symptoms women frequently experience. But to fully appreciate the differences, a general knowledge of how the heart works in all of us is needed.

HOW THE BEAT GOES ON

It's staggering when you stop to think about it. Almost from the time of conception until you draw your last breath, the heart beats *continuously*—dozens of times every single minute—in order to pump 4,300 gallons of blood each day to every organ and tissue in your body. By the time an 85-year-old woman dies, her heart has beaten an estimated 2,680,560,000, or 2.68 billion times.

The mechanism that keeps the heart pumping blood through the 100,000 miles of blood vessels in each of us (enough to circle the earth more than four times) is intricate, elegant, and astounding almost beyond words.

The heart itself is made of muscle that squeezes in upon itself, or contracts, with every beat in order to push blood all the way down to your toes and up to your brain. The muscle is tightly bound in layers that form each of the heart's four chambers: the right atrium, the right ventricle, the left atrium, and the left ventricle.

The Heart

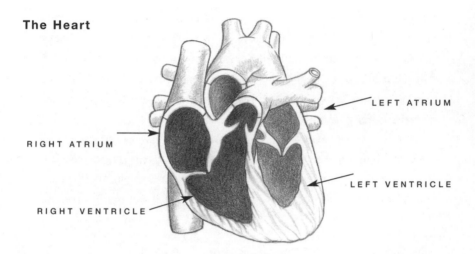

Blood is pumped from the heart to the rest of the body directly from the left ventricle. When the layers of muscle making up the left ventricle contract, the resulting pressure is enough to push blood out of that chamber and then to all the body's arteries—blood vessels that carry blood *away* from the heart.

After the blood passes through all the arteries, it proceeds to the body's 10 billion capillaries. These tiny blood vessels are wide enough for only a single blood cell to pass at any one time. The advantage is that lots of very narrow blood tubules create an extremely large surface area through which oxygen and nutrients can be dropped off to all the cells that compose the various organs and other tissues making up the body. At the same time, carbon dioxide and other waste products are picked up.

From the capillaries, the blood flows to the veins—the vessels that carry blood *back* to the heart.

The Blood Pressure Connection

The pressure occurring at the peak of each heartbeat, when blood is pushed out to the entire body, is called *systolic pressure,* which is the first—and higher—number in a blood pressure reading.

Once the heart has pumped blood into the arteries and is between beats, blood pressure is at its lowest; no extra force is being exerted. That minimum pressure is called *diastolic pressure,* the second number in a blood pressure reading. Diastolic pressure, even when high, is always going to be a lower number than systolic pressure. That's because the pressure of blood against artery walls when the heart muscle first contracts is higher than the pressure in the tubes once the contraction is over and the blood being forced out of the heart has already done a fair amount of its traveling.

What numbers constitute high blood pressure, or hypertension (usually diagnosed with a cuff around your upper arm at routine doctor's visits)? Normal blood pressure? The cutoff points have recently been made more strict with evidence that lower blood pressure is more protective.

Blood pressure	Old classification	New classification (as of 2003)
<120/80 (mm/Hg)*	optimal	normal
120–129/80–84	normal	prehypertension
130–139/85–89	borderline	prehypertension
>140/90	hypertension	hypertension

* mm/Hg stands for millimeters of mercury, meaning the pressure is equivalent to the amount of pressure needed to drive a column of mercury up a tube of a specified width.

Once the blood returns to the heart, it enters through the right atrium (which houses the heart's natural pacemaker). From there it's pumped to the right ventricle. At that point, blood leaves the heart once again, this time for a short trip through the lungs. In the lungs, blood drops off carbon dioxide—a by-product of metabolism—and becomes replenished with oxygen that you've just breathed in. Then it flows into the heart's left atrium and from there to the left ventricle, where the whole process begins anew.

Take Your Resting Pulse

Your pulse, or heart rate, like your blood pressure, is an important indicator of how well your cardiovascular system is doing. Generally speaking, a low resting pulse—closer to, say, 55 beats per minute or lower rather than 70 or higher—indicates that your heart can pump more efficiently. That is, it can pump more blood with each beat and thereby transport plenty of oxygen and nutrients to all the cells of the body with less work.

How can you lower your pulse rate? Through regular exercise. Challenging the heart through aerobic exercise such as brisk walking, running, bicycling, or swimming helps it to beat more efficiently. An elite athlete's resting heart rate can be as low as 30.

To find your resting pulse rate, first thing in the morning before you get out of bed, lightly put your fingers on an artery and count for 30 seconds. Then multiply by two since pulse rate is expressed in beats per minute. Most women can find an artery in either their wrist or their neck because the arteries in those spots are closest to the skin's surface. Beats are felt during the momentary increase in pressure that occurs as the heart muscle contracts. (To find your pulse rate during *exercise,* see the illustration and instructions on page 112.)

Of course, the many parts of this cycle are going on simultaneously. At the same time that deoxygenated blood is flowing through the veins back toward the heart, oxygen-rich blood is headed for the heart from the lungs. Blood is always leaving and approaching the heart at the same time.

When Something Goes Wrong

A system of valves within the heart makes sure blood doesn't flow in the wrong direction. For instance, the *tricuspid valve* separating the upper right chamber from the lower right chamber makes sure blood is always going from the atrium to the ventricle. Similarly, the *bicuspid,* or mitral, valve separates the upper and lower chambers of the left side of the heart. If the valve

The Cardiovascular System

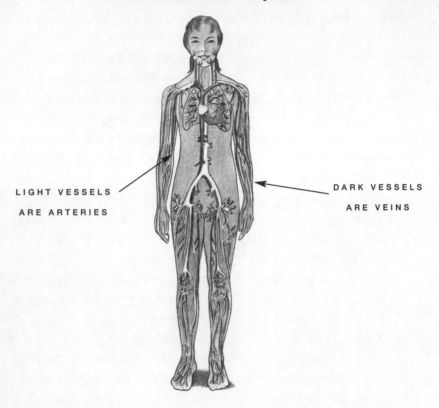

LIGHT VESSELS
ARE ARTERIES

DARK VESSELS
ARE VEINS

does not close completely and there's backward leakage, it's heard with a stethoscope as a *murmur*. Too much backward leakage, and the valve may have to be repaired or even replaced.

But that kind of heart problem is very rare. It's not what most women need to be concerned about. The more common problem has to do with blood flow through the vessels that nourish the heart muscle. Consider that as blood is pumped away from the heart into arteries that bring it to all the organs and tissues of the body, it is also pumped into arteries that nourish the heart muscle itself. After all, the heart muscle, like all other body tissues, needs to have a constant supply of oxygen and nutrients delivered by the blood. And that blood does not come directly from the heart's four chambers but, as with any other organ, from arteries. These arteries are on the outer surface of the heart.

The arteries that bring blood to the heart muscle are referred to as coronary arteries. If any of them become narrowed or partly blocked, not enough oxygen will reach the heart muscle, interfering with function. This happens when cholesterol-rich plaque builds up in them, impeding blood flow, and it's called *coronary heart disease.* (A more general term for blocked arteries is *atherosclerosis,* from the Greek *athero*—gruel or paste—and *sclerosis*—hardness.)

But heart disease is not necessarily just a "plumbing" problem. Blood flow can also be impeded as an indirect result of inflammation. When an atherosclerotic artery becomes inflamed, plaque becomes unstable and can rupture, precipitating the formation of a blood clot—and a subsequent heart attack or stroke.

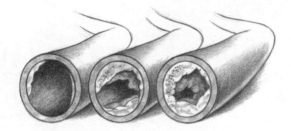

The Progression of Atherosclerosis

The left vessel is relatively free of plaque. The right vessel has advanced plaque and is much more likely to result in blocked blood flow.

Barring an out-and-out coronary event, the heart muscle's blood oxygen deprivation may be felt as *angina*—chest pain or discomfort, perhaps accompanied by pain in the shoulders, arms, neck, jaw, or back. Sometimes angina may be felt on exertion, for example, while hurrying to catch a plane, carrying groceries in from the car, or vacuuming. In such cases, it is known as stable angina. More concerning is unstable angina. The symptoms occur at rest, which suggests that even without exertion, not enough oxygen is getting to the heart muscle. Recently, it has become apparent that in women in particular, angina may also manifest itself simply as fatigue or feeling "not quite right."

Angina and heart attacks occur on a continuum. If the plaque buildup sufficiently narrows a coronary artery, or if even a small amount of plaque made unstable by inflammation causes the formation of a blood clot, most or all blood flow will be cut off and a heart attack, or *myocardial infarction,* can occur. Blood clots can form anywhere in the body, especially if the blood vessels are inflamed, and then travel to—and get stuck in—a coronary artery, or they can form right in a coronary artery itself, causing the abrupt cessation of blood flow. Of course, the more narrowed an artery becomes by plaque, or the more inflammation that is present, the more likely that a clot will block off blood flow.

How Does Plaque Form?

Plaque, which narrows arteries and contributes to the formation of clots, both of which can lead to heart attacks, is made primarily of cholesterol. The majority of cholesterol comes straight from the blood circulating through the body, either directly or indirectly from what is called "bad" LDL-cholesterol, which is why it's so important to keep down LDL-cholesterol levels in the blood.

One way cholesterol is prevented from accumulating in arteries has to do with "good" HDL-cholesterol. How HDL-cholesterol works is complicated, but to oversimplify for a moment, consider that both LDL- and HDL-cholesterol are made from cholesterol and protein. However, the kind of protein in each is different. The protein that is part of LDL-cholesterol causes it to be deposited as plaque on blood vessel walls. The protein that helps make up HDL-cholesterol, on the other hand, enables cholesterol to be picked up from blood vessel walls and carried to the liver via a process called *reverse cholesterol transport.*

The liver, in turn, rids the body of cholesterol in a number of ways. For instance, it can use the cholesterol to make bile acids, which are necessary for digestion. Or it can secrete cholesterol directly into the small intestine to be eliminated from the body.

When Your Brain *Doesn't Get Enough Blood*

The same principle that applies to arteries nourishing the heart also applies to narrowing of the carotid (kah-ROT-id) arteries, the main arteries in the neck that supply blood to the brain. Such blockage is called *carotid artery stenosis,* and the result in this case can be a brain attack, more commonly known as a stroke.

There are actually two kinds of strokes. About 80 percent are ischemic strokes, in which a clot lodges in either the carotid artery or a smaller artery branching out from it. The result is that part of the brain does not get adequate blood; hence, there's an inadequate supply of oxygen, which can kill brain cells. How such a stroke plays out is highly variable, depending on which part of the brain is affected, how large the affected brain region is, and for how long the vessel is blocked. Some people have TIAs, or transient ischemic attacks—greatly diminished blood flow that lasts only a couple of minutes and has no long-term effects (although people who have them are at much higher risk for more serious strokes later). At the other extreme are massive ischemic strokes, which cause paralysis, difficulty speaking, and potentially death.

The other 20 percent of strokes are hemorrhagic strokes—hemorrhaging, or bleeding, into the brain from one of the brain's blood vessels. This type also leads to variable consequences, depending on the brain region affected and the severity of the bleeding. High blood pressure is a major risk factor for hemorrhagic stroke.

Other possible problems (which, unlike blocked arteries, are not always directly affected by lifestyle) include aneurysms, arrhythmias, atrial fibrillation, congestive heart failure, and peripheral vascular disease. For definitions, consult the glossary.

HEART DISEASE'S FEMININE TOUCH

With men, often the first sign of heart disease is a heart attack itself, or at least a distinct tightening or squeezing in the chest upon exertion. Women's first warning signs are often much more subtle: shortness of breath or fatigue when engaging in activities that used to be easy, or even a feeling of mild indigestion. Sometimes there's *diffuse* chest pain. But in one study of 515 women who had had heart attacks, 43 percent said they never experi-

hest discomfort whatsoever; 95 percent, on the other hand, expe-
atively vague symptoms such as fatigue and sleeplessness up to a
ore they were struck.

The male-female differences go deeper than just the symptoms. There are differences in the blood vessels themselves. Women's arteries tend to be smaller than men's. Therefore, if a woman has to undergo bypass surgery, which is a rerouting of blood via insertion of a healthy blood vessel to bypass one that is blocked or nearly blocked, the operation is more difficult and more risky. Perhaps that's one of the reasons that in a review of more than 300,000 people undergoing bypass surgery, the death rate was higher in women.

Women's Hearts React Differently to Emotions

It's not just physical differences that make women's hearts different from men's. Feelings play out differently, too. As you may have heard and could probably intuit even if you haven't, men with type-A personalities are more likely than other men to die after a heart attack, at least according to preliminary research. The stress, anger, and impatience apparently do them in. What's not so commonly known is that women appear more likely to die after a heart attack if they *don't* show their anger, and instead react slowly to negative events, suppressing unpleasant emotions such as agitation during stressful times. In the well-known Framingham Heart Study, women who reported suppressing their anger experienced the highest rate of first heart attacks.

We suspect that there must be a happy middle ground—not flying off the handle at every opportunity but not keeping everything bottled up inside, either.

Isolation may be bad for women's hearts as well. In primate research, being socially isolated and having limited freedom of movement was correlated with greater heart disease among females. And female monkeys housed alone have been found to suffer more extensive atherosclerosis than their counterparts housed in social groups.

But what makes women's hearts *most* unlike men's is not their heart disease symptoms, nor the apparatus that makes up their cardiovascular systems, nor the way their hearts react to emotional stress or social situations. It's the way their hearts are *perceived*—both by physicians and by women themselves.

WOMEN'S HEARTS UNDERATTENDED BY THE MEDICAL COMMUNITY

Bypass surgery may be trickier to perform on women's narrower arteries, but an even bigger problem is that fewer women who need bypasses ever get them. There continues to linger a perception on the part of the health care community that heart disease is a man's illness. In one Canadian study of more than 30,000 people who had had either a heart attack or unstable angina, women were 30 percent less likely than men to undergo revascularization—procedures to open up blocked blood vessels. In fact, women undergo intensive treatment for heart disease much less frequently than men with symptoms of the same severity. Sometimes a man with *less* severe symptoms than a woman will still be more likely to get more intensive treatment. When researchers at the Tufts–New England Medical Center conducted a study of 889 patients with acute angina, they found that only 2 percent were mistakenly discharged from hospital emergency departments around the country. But the percentage for women under age 55 was much greater. They were *seven* times more likely not to be admitted straight from the emergency room than were people in other groups.

Women's seemingly vague symptoms continue not to be recognized as frequently as men's for the heart attacks they can turn out to be. Even the way physicians manage chest pain itself has been shown to be influenced by the gender of the patient. As you'll see in a later chapter, in some cases a woman's symptoms have to be extreme before her heart disease is fully recognized for what it is.

When women *are* finally treated for cardiovascular problems, it's often very late in their disease development and therefore less likely to be helpful. For instance, women who do undergo bypass surgery typically are sicker and older than their male counterparts. Due to late detection and intervention, their heart disease is more advanced, and therefore more severe.

It's not just *treatment* that's lacking for women. So are *evaluation* and diagnostic procedures. Women who have had a heart attack are less likely than male heart attack patients to undergo cardiac catheterization, a procedure that analyzes blood flow in the arteries leading to the heart in order to ascertain the location and extent of the damage. Women physicians prescribe the test to their female patients just as infrequently as male doctors do, according to a study that looked at the records of 104,000 Medicare heart patients.

Women are also less likely to undergo the standard treadmill test that helps ascertain heart disease risk. Think about it: When the treadmill test comes to mind, we tend to envision a man huffing and puffing to exhaustion.

But a woman's level of fitness, measured by a standardized treadmill exercise test, might be even more predictive of whether she'll die than a man is. In a 2003 study conducted at Chicago's Rush Institute, researchers followed 5,700 women who had had their exercise capacity assessed on treadmills. Eight years later, those who were not able to work up to walking at least 2.5 miles per hour on an incline with a 12 percent grade (equivalent to a very steep hill) were almost twice as likely to die as those who could. Women who couldn't progress even to 1.7 miles an hour on a 10 percent incline (still a rather steep hill) were three times as likely to die during that eight-year span. **The results showed physical fitness to be an even more important predictor of death for women than for men—by twofold.** For this reason, we have included a physical fitness test in the next chapter to help you assess your heart disease risk.

WOMEN'S HEARTS UNDERATTENDED BY WOMEN THEMSELVES

If glossing over the state of women's hearts by the medical community isn't enough, women themselves often give their hearts short shrift. In fact, one of the reasons women die more often than men following a heart attack is that they wait longer to go to the hospital when they're having one; hence, more heart muscle has already died by the time they receive treatment.

Women are inclined to ignore or downplay red flags because they don't *expect* to get heart disease, even though it's their number-one killer. They misinterpret their own less-than-clear-cut symptoms. Indeed, while more than *ten times* as many women die of cardiovascular disease than of breast cancer, women think their risk of dying from heart disease is only twice the risk of dying from breast cancer, according to one survey. Of even

greater concern, the same survey indicates that only 7 percent of
consider heart disease their greatest problem, whereas 34 percent cit
cancer.

Can Your Daily Routine Provide a Hint About Your Heart Disease Risk?

Men often don't get clues that a heart attack is in the offing. They feel absolutely fine one moment and are laid low the next. Women have an advantage in that regard. If a woman has to slow down to get tasks done, if she gets
winded doing something that she used to be able to do with ease, if she simply has to stop doing something that's very important to her, it can be a sign
of heart disease or even an impending heart attack. And such early warning
signs—if recognized—can allow a woman to get help before a lot of damage
is done.

Unfortunately, doctors don't tend to ask questions about daily routine
when they assess patients for heart disease. They talk about more intense
kinds of physical activity, like brisk walking or swimming. Also, a doctor may
ask, "Are you having chest pains?" But that question can be misleading. A
woman may answer no simply because she has stopped doing something, or
started doing it more slowly, in order to avoid chest pains. At the same time,
a doctor may *not* ask about symptoms that could be very telling, such as
fatigue or a vague feeling of nausea.

To keep from falling through the cracks before heart disease has gone
too far, all women should periodically ask themselves a series of questions
about their ability to perform routine activities. For instance, many women,
over time, have to modify the way they do things like carry laundry up the
stairs or change the sheets. (Changing bed linens, which research has shown
can take a fair amount of energy, has been marked as the household
task most commonly done differently because of heart disease symptoms.
Women stop for rests more, or do the work more slowly.) So one of the questions should be:

Can I handle housework without difficulty, or has it become more difficult? Do I have to rest in the middle of a chore that I used to be able to sail
through without taking breaks?

Other potential questions:

- Have I stopped doing yardwork and gardening as rigorously as I used to?
- Have I developed a habit of letting things accumulate at the bottom of the stairs so I only have to make one trip upstairs each day?
- Do I now check my bags before boarding a flight because it has become too hard to walk through the airport with them?
- Has it gotten harder for me to carry things in from the car?

If the answers to these and other questions related to your daily habits are yes, it does not necessarily mean you have heart disease. There are lots of reasons a woman might not be able to do something as well as she used to: arthritis pain, for instance, or back trouble, or just plain old slowing down with aging. But a decline in ability to do chores that are very important to you or that you need to complete as a matter of course should serve as a signal that it's time to make a doctor's appointment.

TURNING THE TIDE

Lack of attention to the possibility of heart disease also means lack of attention to prevention. When you think of a heart attack victim, you probably think of an overweight man, perhaps a smoker, who doesn't get any exercise and doesn't watch what he eats. But take a look at the numbers. An estimated 34 percent of all women in America are overweight, and another 30 percent are obese. Twenty-five percent of women report that they do no regular physical activity. (That number goes up as women age.) Twenty-two million American women smoke. The prevalence of high blood pressure, another major heart disease risk factor, is *rising* in women but not in men—no doubt at least in part because women are getting heavier. In other words, women fit the heart attack profile, too.

The silver lining in all this is that women can lower their heart disease risk—both by living more healthfully and by becoming more attuned to possible signs of heart trouble. Armed with that greater awareness, a woman is in a much better position to partner with her doctor both to avoid heart disease and, if need be, to identify it in its early stages so that it can be tended to before any major damage is done. In the chapters that follow, you'll learn how.

CHAPTER 3

Take the Test to Learn Your Risk

◆

I kind of suspected *high blood pressure was coming. My sister, who is twelve years younger than I am, has had high blood pressure since she was in her thirties. And both my mother and father have it. I wasn't too concerned about my cholesterol, however. It had always been fine. In fact, I had gotten a little cocky about it, not being as careful about eating right and all that (although I was still thin). But when my physician finally checked it again after several years, it had gone way up.*

—ANNE

H ow likely are you to suffer a heart attack, stroke, or other coronary "event" in the next ten years? Do you have a 10 percent chance? Twenty percent? Greater than 20 percent?

These are not theoretical questions. Every single woman, particularly by age 40, should know her risk for developing cardiovascular disease so that she can develop an appropriate game plan for preventing it. There's an imperative for preventing that first heart attack, stroke, or other coronary complication. The rate of first "events" that are disabling, and even fatal, is very high. Fifty percent of people having a heart attack die before they ever get to the hospital.

Maybe you assume you're at low risk and therefore don't need to be concerned. But almost 40 percent of women, as well as men, in the United States are at *moderate* risk, meaning they have an elevated chance of experiencing a heart attack or other cardiovascular-related calamity that could prove deadly. They need to take some specific steps to protect themselves. Unfortunately, many of them—perhaps the majority—don't know it, because they don't know how to assess their own risk for heart disease, or because they have never been concerned about it.

Granted, in some cases their doctors may know it, assigning them a risk score periodically. But *you* should be aware of it, too. One reason is that the better informed you are, the more committed you'll be to making the changes necessary to lower your chances of having a heart attack or stroke. At least as important, a lot of people fall through cracks in the medical system. Either they aren't treated aggressively enough, or they're treated *too* aggressively, being slapped with a drug prescription before they've had a chance to see if changes in diet and physical activity patterns alone are enough to improve heart health. Keeping apprised of your risk level will help you to work *with* your doctor by allowing you to keep track of whether you're following the *right* plan for protecting your heart.

PUTTING A NUMBER TO IT

Exactly how do you quantify your heart disease risk? There's a scoring system put out by the National Heart, Lung, and Blood Institute that's often used as an initial screening tool. Fortunately, it's extremely easy to tally up, requiring that you answer only five questions about yourself (other than your gender): your age, total blood cholesterol, smoking status, HDL-cholesterol level ("good" cholesterol), and systolic blood pressure (that first number in a blood pressure reading).

Obviously, you'll need to get a couple of these answers during a physical at your doctor's office. If you've had a physical within the last two years that also included blood work and a blood pressure reading, you can call the doctor's office for the numbers. If more time than that has gone by, you should still call the doctor's office—to make an appointment. (Before you read on, write a note to yourself in the margin of this page or on a slip of paper as a reminder to phone your physician's office, if necessary.)

The doctor will draw blood to measure your total and HDL-cholesterol and, in many cases, your LDL-cholesterol level as well. If the numbers are outside the desirable range, you will probably be asked to come back and have blood drawn after an overnight fast to confirm the reading. At that time, the doctor will also tell the lab to check your LDL-cholesterol (if it wasn't previously measured) and your blood triglyceride level, which can be correctly determined only after a fast. (See the box on page 32 for more on triglycerides.)

You'll see below that each answer to the five questions is assigned a certain value. Add the total points for your five answers, then match the sum to your ten-year risk. As the chart makes clear, if your point total falls below 20, your coronary heart disease risk is below 10 percent, which means it's low. If your point total runs between 20 and 22, your coronary heart disease risk is between 10 and 20 percent, which means it's moderate. And a score of 23 or higher means your chance of suffering from heart disease or any of its complications over the next ten years is greater than 20 percent—high. (*Your risk is automatically considered greater than 20 percent if you already have heart disease or diabetes, no matter what your score on these five questions.*)

1. Age	Points	Age	Points
20–34	-7	55–59	8
35–39	-3	60-64	10
40–44	0	65-69	12
45–49	3	70-74	14
50–54	6	75 and up	16

2. Total Cholesterol	Age				
(milligrams per deciliter of blood)	20–39	40–49	50–59	60–69	70–79
	Points				
Less than 160	0	0	0	0	0
160–199	4	3	2	1	1
200–239	8	6	4	2	1
240–279	11	8	5	3	2
At or greater than 280	13	10	7	4	2

3. Smoking History	Age				
	20–39	40–49	50–59	60–69	70–79
	Points				
Nonsmoker	0	0	0	0	0
Smoker	9	7	4	2	1

4. HDL-Cholesterol

(milligrams per deciliter of blood)	Points
60 or above	-1
50–59	0
40–49	1
Less than 40	2

5. Systolic Blood Pressure	If Untreated	If Treated
Less than 120	0	0
120–129	1	3
130–139	2	4
140–159	3	5
At least 160	4	6

YOUR TOTAL POINTS: _____

Point Total	Your Ten–Year Risk	
	(% chance of experiencing a heart attack)	
Less than 9	Less than 1%	Low Risk
9–12	1	Low Risk
13–14	2	Low Risk
15	3	Low Risk

Point Total	Your Ten–Year Risk	
	(% chance of experiencing a heart attack)	
16	4	Low Risk
17	5	Low Risk
18	6	Low Risk
19	8	Low Risk
20	11	Moderate Risk
21	14	Moderate Risk
22	17	Moderate Risk
23	22	High Risk
24	27	High Risk
25 or more	At least 30%	High Risk

How high your risk is dictates just how aggressive you should be in your heart disease prevention efforts. For instance, if it's less than 10 percent, and therefore low, there's probably not much you need to alter in your current lifestyle to keep heart disease at bay. But if your chance of suffering a heart attack or related problem over the next ten years is at least 20 percent, or high, you'll need to take more intensive measures to get it down, by making more of an effort to lose some excess weight, if need be, in addition to eating a more healthful diet in general and exercising appropriately. In addition, your physician will likely start you on a drug regimen. For someone at high risk, lifestyle and medications together can be a powerful deterrent of cardiovascular events.

If you're at moderate risk for having a heart attack or a related event in the next ten years, 10 to 20 percent, the intensity of your lifestyle efforts and whether you should take a drug will be a judgment call.

What About LDL-Cholesterol?

Your level of LDL-cholesterol presently isn't used to calculate your ten-year heart disease risk, but your risk score dictates, in part, what your LDL-cholesterol level should be. Indeed, there may be nothing more important you can do than to keep down your LDL-cholesterol.

To determine the LDL-cholesterol that is right for you, you also need to tally how many risk factors you have; the more you have, the higher your risk. The risk factors that are especially applicable to *women* (we know you have already factored in some of them):

- Cigarette smoking
- High blood pressure (at or greater than 140/90 without medication)
- Low HDL-cholesterol (less than 50 mg/dl)
- Family history of premature heart disease (under age 65 in a female first-degree relative and under age 55 in a male first-degree relative)
- Age (at least 55)

People at low risk for heart disease, as indicated by your point score and your number of risk factors, are considered healthier with higher levels of LDL-cholesterol in their blood than people at moderate or high risk. Simply put, they have more wiggle room for higher LDL-cholesterol levels.

Level of Risk (from pages 27–28)	LDL-Cholesterol Goal (milligrams per deciliter of blood)
10-year risk below 10% + 0–1 risk factor	160 or lower
10-year risk below 10% + 2 or more risk factors	130 or lower
10-year risk of 10–20% + 2 or more risk factors	130 or lower (Your physician may set an LDL goal closer to 100)
10-year risk of 20% or higher	100 or lower (Your physician may set an LDL goal closer to 70)

Note: You can subtract one risk factor from the total if your HDL-cholesterol is above 60 mg/dl.

Do You Have Metabolic Syndrome?

While keeping LDL-cholesterol appropriately low is the most critical step for warding off a heart attack or other cardiovascular event, it's also important to determine whether you have something called *metabolic syndrome*—and to get treatment if you do. Metabolic syndrome in itself raises the chances of heart disease, independently of LDL-cholesterol levels.

How do you determine whether you have metabolic syndrome? You can't *feel* it; there are no symptoms. Rather, it's a cluster of risk factors. If, with your doctor, you determine that you have at least three out of the following risk factors, you've got it.

- Abdominal obesity (waist circumference greater than 35 inches)*
- High triglycerides (at least 150 milligrams per deciliter of blood)
- Low HDL-cholesterol (less than 50 milligrams per deciliter of blood)*
- High blood pressure (at least 130/85)
- High fasting glucose, or blood sugar, which is a precursor to diabetes (at least 110 milligrams per deciliter of blood)

Management of metabolic syndrome, which occurs as frequently in postmenopausal women as in men, includes a combination of weight loss, dietary modification, and increased physical activity and, in some cases, medications. These approaches will also reduce LDL-cholesterol in someone who has high levels.

People with metabolic syndrome must not go on a very low-fat diet, which could actually exacerbate the condition by increasing triglyceride levels, as we will explain shortly.

The numbers apply specifically to women.

Other Important Factors to Consider

You may be wondering why some other important numbers aren't part of the National Heart, Lung, and Blood Institute's scoring system: your weight, for instance, or the amount of time you spend in moderately vigorous physical activity. Part of the reason is that this self-assessment measures your *primary* risk factors for heart disease. For example, your weight certainly influences your risk, but it's *secondary*. That is, excess weight is a risk factor because it tends to increase primary risk factors such as blood cholesterol, blood pressure, and elevated fasting glucose. Indeed, women who are even only a little bit overweight can be at as much as a sevenfold increased risk for heart disease compared to their thinner counterparts, according to findings from Harvard's Nurses' Health Study. Still, excess weight in and of itself does not increase your chances of having a heart attack or stroke. It's the high cholesterol, hypertension, and high fasting blood glucose levels that do that.

There are other things that influence risk secondarily that are also worth considering. For instance, both the Iowa Women's Study and the Nurses' Health Study, which combined follow some 150,000 women, have reported that women who eat diets with more daily servings of whole grains, fruits, and vegetables than other women are at decreased risk for developing heart disease. It's hard to tease out exactly how that dietary pattern works. We do know that whole grains and produce contain fiber, which can play a role in lowering blood cholesterol. Diets that are high in fiber also tend to be relatively low in calories. Therefore, this kind of eating pattern can help keep down weight. It also helps ward off diabetes, which is a very big heart disease risk in itself, especially in women. Finally, healthful diets rich in vegetables, fruits, and whole grains leave less room for foods like pastries, ice cream, cookies, candy, and fatty cuts of meat, all of which can negatively influence blood cholesterol and thereby raise heart disease risk.

Considering Triglycerides

One of the most hotly debated questions in the cardiovascular field is how important the level of triglycerides in your blood is for estimating your heart disease risk. One study published several years ago in the *Archives of Internal Medicine* found that triglyceride levels in women (but not in men) were useful for estimating heart disease risk. But the number of women observed was too small to draw any conclusions with confidence, and the issue is not straightforward in the first place.

One of the reasons it's not at all clear whether high triglyceride levels provide additional information about disease risk is that in the majority of cases, when triglycerides are high, HDL-cholesterol is low, and vice versa. Even more to the point for women actively trying to lower their chance for heart disease is that the approach to lowering high triglyceride levels overlaps with that for raising HDL-cholesterol levels—lose excess weight and increase physical activity.

If you're overweight and lose more than 10 percent of your body weight, you may be able to lower your triglycerides by as much as 30 to 40 percent at the same time that you raise HDL-cholesterol. And there is preliminary evidence that if you become more physically active, you can lower triglycerides by as much as 10 percent and again, raise HDL-cholesterol.

Put another way, screening for triglycerides may be something of a moot point. You should already be doing what it takes to keep those levels down. The only thing some women with high triglycerides may be advised to do in addition to taking the other lifestyle steps is cut down *a little* on carbohydrates (fewer cakes, cookies, pasta, and white bread) and replace the lost calories with *a little* unsaturated fat, such as vegetable oil or the fat in fish. A very low-fat diet can raise triglycerides dramatically in some women.

Triglyceride Categories (which must be assessed via a blood test
taken after an overnight fast)

Normal:	less than 150 (milligrams per deciliter of blood)
Borderline high:	150–199
High:	200–499
Very high:	500 or more

THE FITNESS FACTOR

As far as physical activity level, a sedentary lifestyle is considered an important risk factor for heart disease. It directly influences a woman's chances of having a heart attack or stroke down the line. One reason it's not part of the risk scoring system is that in certain ways, it's hard to measure exactly the degree to which fitness impacts heart disease risk. We know that being active reduces blood pressure and blood glucose, improves circulation and HDL-cholesterol levels, and helps promote weight control, for instance, but not all the connections on a biological level have been fully sorted out. Still, it has become clear that physical inactivity, in conjunction with a poor diet, is about to eclipse tobacco as the leading cause of death in the United States.

For that reason we feel it's very important for you to take a fitness assessment in addition to the assessment at the beginning of this chapter. It will give you at least some indication of whether your current fitness level is decreasing your heart disease risk or contributing to it. You can return to this assessment after the physical activity program outlined in chapter 6 becomes a habit. Every three months is reasonable for monitoring your progress. You may be surprised at the positive changes.

How Fit Are You?

If you can comfortably walk a mile, take this simple test to estimate your aerobic fitness: walk for 12 minutes as fast as you can. Over the coming weeks and months, repeat the test to track your fitness progress.

This assessment tool was developed by colleagues of ours at the Cooper Institute in Dallas. They tested hundreds of women (and men) and came up with the chart on page 35, which has been shown to compare very well for accuracy to the numbers generated by more technical physical fitness assessment procedures.

Take the Cooper Test

Step 1:   Take the Par-Q questionnaire on page 104 to see if you need to check with your doctor before taking the test.

Step 2:   Find a local track you have permission to use, such as at a high school, college, or community center, and find out how many laps equal a mile.

Step 3:   Select a day when the weather is good. Dress in comfortable clothes and athletic shoes. Bring along a stopwatch—or a watch with big hands and an easy-to-read face—plus a pencil and paper.

Step 4:   Before the test, warm up for five minutes by walking at a moderate pace.

Step 5:   Start the stopwatch and walk as fast as you can *for 12 minutes.* If you regularly run or jog, you may do so for all or part of the test.

Step 6:   Note the number of laps around the track you complete, including any partial distance you cover during the final lap, before the 12 minutes are up.

Step 7:   Slow your pace and cool down by walking slowly for five minutes.

Step 8:   Write down the number of times you went around the track, including the partial distance of the final lap. Calculate the distance that you covered. Check the chart to determine your fitness level.

	Cooper Twelve–Minute Walking/Running Test *Distance Covered (in Miles) in Twelve Minutes*					
FITNESS CATEGORY	AGE					
	13–19	20–29	30–39	40–49	50–59	60+
Superior	>1.52	>1.46	>1.40	>1.35	>1.31	>1.19
Excellent	1.44–1.51	1.35–1.45	1.30–1.39	1.25–1.35	1.19–1.30	1.10–1.18
Good	1.30–1.43	1.23–1.34	1.19–1.29	1.12–1.24	1.06–1.18	.99–1.09
Fair	1.19–1.29	1.12–1.22	1.06–1.18	.99–1.11	.94–1.05	.87–.98
Poor	1.00–1.18	.96–1.11	.95–1.05	.88–.98	.84–.93	.78–.86
Very Poor	<1.0	<.96	<.94	<.88	<.84	<.78
	Laps covered: _____ Distance in miles: _____ Your age: _____ Determine your fitness level: _____					

If you fall into the "Excellent" or "Superior" category, congratulate yourself; fitness-wise, you are at a relatively low risk for heart disease. That doesn't mean that you don't need to exercise (or control and improve other risk factors). It means you have a good fitness foundation from which to proceed. If you are in the "Good" category, there is room for improvement, and your health will benefit if you become more fit. If you score "Fair" or lower, your heart is incontrovertibly being compromised by your fitness level. The good news is that by following the *Strong Women, Strong Hearts* exercise program, outlined in chapter 6, your fitness level will soar—and so will your heart health.

EMERGING RISK FACTORS

The nature of heart disease research is such that new risk factors are being discovered all the time. It is not yet clear how powerfully they influence the chances of having a heart attack or stroke, but scientists are busy determining whether physicians should be ordering lab tests for some of them. Here's a rundown.

High-Sensitivity C-Reactive Protein

If you're at moderate risk for heart disease—you scored a 10 to 20 percent chance of suffering a cardiovascular event in the next ten years—you should talk to your doctor about whether it's advisable to get a test for what's known as high-sensitivity C-reactive protein, or CRP. The CRP test checks for inflammation in the body, arteries included. While a high level of cholesterol means there is probably a buildup of plaque in the arteries that impedes the flow of blood (at least in part), a high CRP score means there's a chance that there's a lot of *inflammation* in the arteries. And that inflammation, which can be brought on by such factors as injury to blood vessel walls, cigarette smoking, and high blood pressure, can cause any of the plaque present to potentially rupture—triggering clots that might bring on a heart attack or stroke.

The test is not advised for people at low risk for heart disease because a high number wouldn't alter the lifestyle recommendations. A CRP test also isn't recommended for people at high risk because they should already be receiving aggressive treatment—making very intensive efforts with their diet and physical activity patterns and, if necessary, taking drugs to bring down their cholesterol level or treat other risk factors. But for patients at moderate risk for whom doctors are undecided about prescribing drugs, the outcome of the CRP test could help them make up their minds.

Note: While you should definitely have your CRP tested if your doctor recommends it, some of the latest reports question its value in predicting heart disease risk. One reason is that because the test signifies inflammation anywhere in the body, not just the arteries, a high value could be a false alarm. Even someone with a minor cold or a flare-up due to an infection can have an elevated level. In addition, there is some evidence that the test as a whole doesn't hold up nearly as strongly as a predictive measure for heart disease in women as in men. Thus, CRP levels should be interpreted very cautiously.

Homocysteine

Some evidence suggests that high blood levels of homocysteine (ho-mo-CIS-teen), a metabolic product of an amino acid found in proteins, is a marker for heart disease. Homocysteine builds up not because someone eats too much protein but for a variety of other reasons, including a low intake of certain B vitamins.

Researchers suspect that excess homocysteine may damage the lining of blood vessels or trigger the growth of cells that help form fatty deposits, namely plaque, on artery walls. It may also accelerate artery damage by encouraging the breakdown of LDL-cholesterol within plaque, adding to damage that results in the arteries becoming harder and less supple.

But it's not proven. It may be that homocysteine doesn't *cause* artery damage but, rather, is the *result* of it. If that's the case, lowering homocysteine in the blood won't actually reduce the risk for developing heart disease. Scientists are still working out cause and effect.

Given the uncertainties, physicians are divided on whether they should test for homocysteine routinely. On the plus side, the test is relatively inexpensive, usually running somewhere between $25 and $50. On the minus side, it's another number that can cause anxiety when, in fact, it may not have any predictive value. (A number above 12—micromoles per liter of blood—is generally considered high.)

The good news is that, for most people, reducing homocysteine levels in the blood is not difficult. Colleagues of ours at Tufts have helped demonstrate that you just have to make sure to eat enough of the following three B vitamins: folate, B_6, and B_{12}. Our eating plan in chapter 5 will ensure that you do.

Small, Dense LDL

It's not just knowing how much LDL-cholesterol you have that's important. It's also knowing the *size* of the LDL particles, some researchers believe. The smaller the LDL particles, the denser they are and the heavier for their size.

That means they are most likely to remain in your bloodstream and eventually be taken up by cells that add to plaque more readily than large, "puffy" LDL particles.

It's not clear who are the best candidates for small dense LDL screening. Furthermore, the test is expensive (about $225), few health insurance companies will reimburse for it, and few laboratories can do it in-house. Just as important, the medical community is not convinced that it should be a standard part of anyone's diagnostic care. More to the point, your physician most likely would not use the information to treat you differently than if she/he did not have the information. It's still too new, particularly given the fact that we don't yet know how prominently small dense LDL figures in heart disease risk in the majority of women. Additionally, it is not clear *how* to shift the balance from small dense to large LDL. Any recommendation would be the same as what would be given to reduce elevated LDL-cholesterol levels.

ApoE4

Every single person has a gene called apoE on chromosome number 19. About 15 percent of the population has a form of that gene, or mutation, called apoE4 (as opposed to the most common form, apoE3, or a rarer form, apoE2), which makes them particularly prone to high blood cholesterol if they eat a high-fat diet—and puts them at higher risk of developing heart disease. The flip side is that individuals with the apoE4 mutation are more likely to respond to changes in their diets.

The reality is, genetic testing isn't yet part of routine medical exams; it would be too expensive at this point to do on a patient-by-patient basis. So very few people know which form of the apoE gene they have. But not too many years down the line, it is expected that efficient, inexpensive ways to sequence people's genes will be developed, which will allow doctors (and their patients!) to know who has to be more careful about limiting saturated fat in the diet, keeping down their weight, and so on.

Lipoprotein Associated Phospholipase A2 (Lp-PLA2)

An enzyme known as Lp-PLA2 is released by white blood cells in response to inflammation. It travels through the bloodstream by piggybacking onto LDL

particles, causing the release of material from the particles that c̲
plaque on the artery walls more likely to rupture and trigger a blood
can lead to a heart attack.

Screening for Lp-PLA2 might be useful as a predictor of heart disease risk in people with low LDL levels. Theoretically, if you have low LDL-cholesterol levels, you're at low heart disease risk, but there are plenty of people with low LDL who have heart attacks. It has been observed that a number of them have relatively high concentrations of Lp-PLA2. The thinking is that the more of that enzyme you have, the more likely that even a small amount of LDL-cholesterol in your bloodstream can both trigger plaque growth and the likelihood that the plaque will rupture, causing the formation of an obstructing clot.

The Food and Drug Administration formally approved a lab test for Lp-PLA2 in July 2003. But at this point, whether to screen for the substance or not is at the doctor's discretion. There are no formal recommendations because the value of the screen has yet to be adequately evaluated.

Myeloperoxidase (MPO)

Emerging research suggests that this protein works in similar fashion to Lp-PLA2. It's released in response to inflammation, and its presence has been related to plaque instability, meaning that it is more likely to form a life-threatening clot. But whereas Lp-PLA2 works through LDL-cholesterol particles that then influence plaque, MPO acts more directly on the plaque itself. Screening of MPO has yet to be approved by the Food and Drug Administration.

RISK IS A MOVING TARGET

Knowing your risk for heart disease is critical not only because it lets you know how high your chances are for developing heart disease. As we said earlier, it's also an excellent motivator for making the lifestyle changes necessary to lower your risk. When you can attach a number, or numbers, to something, it makes it more tangible—and easier to set goals for changing that number.

That's what happened with Anne, the woman quoted at the beginning of this chapter, who found out she had high cholesterol. She immediately started making alterations to her diet to help bring her cholesterol down: substituting nonfat creamer for heavy cream in her coffee; switching from regular ice cream (which she ate almost every night) to low-fat ice cream; and so on. Her cholesterol went from "too high" to "desirable." Specifically, her total cholesterol dropped from 227 to 193, and her LDL-cholesterol went from 141 to 121.

Even women who find that their risk is quite low to start with can use such information to keep doing everything right as far as eating healthfully, maintaining a healthy body weight, getting enough exercise, and not smoking. It's much easier to keep risk low than to let it creep up and *then* try to decrease it. Likewise, for women who find their risk is moderate or high, it's much easier to bring down the number: the less time time has passed, the less poor habits have become firmly entrenched, and the less damage has been done to your arteries.

CHAPTER 4

New Insights: Unraveling the Latest Research

❖

If we could give every individual the right amount of nourishment and exercise, not too little and not too much, we would have found the safest way to health.

—HIPPOCRATES, 460–377 B.C.

This is a great time to be a woman who wants to avoid heart disease. It has been more than twenty years since heart disease began to claim more women's lives each year than men's, yet only in the last decade or so has research into women and cardiovascular health gained enough ground so that specific recommendations for our gender could be formed on the basis of scientific findings. The turning point came in early 1993, when the National Institutes of Health *mandated* that half of all human research be conducted on women.

Before that, the basis for most advice to women about how to lower their heart disease risk had to be extrapolated from findings about men. To be fair, in the 1950s and 1960s, it was men who were losing their lives to heart attacks and related events in the prime of life. And even *they* did not have a huge arsenal of lifestyle strategies at their disposal to reduce the risk of heart disease—or stall it if it had already developed.

For instance, as late as the 1960s, the prevailing thought among many was that vigorous exercise might prove dangerous for people at risk for heart disease. And after someone had a heart attack, the advice was to rest—unlike to-day, when the advice is most often to get active again as soon as possible. In-deed, the term "aerobics," which refers to exercises that specifically target the heart and lungs and which everyone now knows, wasn't even coined until the mid-sixties. Until then, the idea of physical activity to protect the heart was limited largely to obscure occupational health studies. In one of them, London bus conductors (all men) who walked up and down the stairs of double-decker buses collecting fares had a lower rate of heart disease deaths than London bus *drivers,* who sat on the job. In another, London postal workers (again, men) with a walking route had a lower level of heart disease than sedentary civil servants—telephonists, executives, and clerks, who sat all day.

Some people still feel that research into stemming heart disease isn't as important for women as it is for men because women tend to develop it later in life, after menopause. But that's only partly true. Yes, if a woman develops heart disease, it tends, on average, to be about ten years later than a man. But in the first direct look at the blood vessels of a large group of young women, researchers have discovered that the fatty streaks and artery-clogging plaque that predispose people to heart attacks and other life-threatening coronary events appear in the blood vessels of girls as young as 15.

The investigators who made this finding were involved in a multicenter study called the Pathobiological Determinants in Youth. Their discovery came during autopsies in which they examined the aortas and coronary ar-teries of young adults who had died from accidents or other untimely causes between the ages of 15 and 34. What they found was that the girls and women had even more extensive amounts of fatty streaks—the beginning of atherosclerotic plaque—than the men. They also found that the presence of *raised* plaque, the type that can start impeding blood flow, increased with age in both women and men. Raised plaque was somewhat more extensive at any given age in men than women, which might help to explain why women ex-hibit heart disease later in life than men do, but women should not necessar-ily take comfort in this. Rather, they should take it as motivation to live more heart healthfully while still young because it means that they have at least as good a chance as men, if not better, of *slowing* the progression of plaque development.

Research is focused not only on youth but on menopause and beyond as well. As we said in chapter 1, recent findings have shown that hormone replacement therapy (HRT), for decades regarded as protective against heart disease after menopause, is actually linked to a small but significant *increase* in heart disease risk. The Women's Health Initiative showed that the chances of suffering a heart attack, stroke, or life-threatening blood clot increase significantly within months of starting HRT.

That doesn't mean HRT is the wrong choice in the short term for every single woman who is suffering from intolerable hot flashes. But it does mean that based on the current evidence, it certainly has no benefit in *reducing* the incidence of heart disease and stroke, and potentially makes them more likely to occur. It can no longer be viewed as an easy, quick fix.

Also driving the need for a better understanding of how to protect women from heart disease is the fact that it is becoming more common as women, along with the rest of the population, get heavier. As indicated in chapter 3, excess body weight raises your risk for developing heart disease by contributing to increases in LDL-cholesterol levels and blood pressure. It also raises the risk for developing diabetes, which, again, leads to a greater risk for heart disease in women than in men.

What follows is a look at the latest research on the diet and exercise factors that form the basis of the *Strong Women, Strong Hearts* program. These findings hold great promise, and when implemented they can help you take control of your heart health for life.

THE DIETARY UNDERPINNINGS

Scientists have been piecing together those elements of the diet that contribute to heart disease and also those that help to prevent it so that, over time, a clear-cut beneficial eating *pattern* has emerged. There is still much to be learned about how to best tweak the diet to make it more heart-healthy, particularly for women. But we know so much more than we did even ten or twenty years ago.

Literally tens of thousands of investigators worldwide have been participating in the research—the best approach, since an accumulated body of evidence corroborated by many independent investigators is the most reliable. Studies conducted in the Cardiovascular Nutrition Laboratory at Tufts, directed by Alice, have made a significant contribution to the scientific findings we have gathered here.

The Fatty Connection

For many years researchers focused on the *amount* of fat in the diet. But now it is clear that the *type* of fat we eat has more to do with our heart disease risk.

Saturated Fat

Even women who have had just a passing interest in nutrition over the years are aware that saturated fat, found in animal foods such as beef, pork, and lamb as well as full-fat dairy products like whole milk and cheese, is the biggest dietary contributor to elevated LDL-cholesterol. Researchers started putting together evidence about saturated fat back in the 1950s, although there were hints even before that. Since then the evidence has accumulated, in both women and men. Specifically, when saturated fat is compared head to head in the diet with unsaturated fat, either monounsaturated or polyunsaturated, LDL-cholesterol levels in the blood are higher, and the risk of developing heart disease is greater.

Studies in which large numbers of people are observed (frequently referred to as epidemiologic studies) have shown that those individuals who eat the most saturated fat are at the highest risk for developing heart disease. Thus, it's important to keep saturated fat intake low—less than 10 percent of calories (the limits are actually for saturated fat and *trans*-fatty acids combined, which we'll discuss shortly). If you found your heart disease risk to be at least 10 percent in chapter 3, then the goal is to keep saturated fat to less than 7 percent of calories.

You don't need to numerically calculate your percentage of calories from saturated fat. As we'll show you in the next chapter, it's considerably easier than that. You just need to think in terms of foods that contain animal fat versus foods that don't and also *how much* of various foods you eat. That will automatically get you to the right percentages. We'll show you, too, that you can limit saturated fat in your diet and still eat terrific-tasting food.

How much lowering of LDL-cholesterol in your bloodstream can you expect from decreasing the saturated fat in your diet? In one study conducted at Tufts's Cardiovascular Nutrition Laboratory, women who switched from

What's Saturated Fat, Monounsaturated Fat, and Polyunsaturated Fat?

Strictly speaking, fats themselves are not saturated, monounsaturated, or polyunsaturated. It's certain *components* of fats—fatty acids—that determine their level of saturation. Without dragging anyone back into high school chemistry class, fatty acids are long chains of carbon atoms joined together by either single or double bonds. Saturated fatty acids have no double bonds, monounsaturated have one double bond, and polyunsaturated have two or more.

The number of double bonds is critical. Why? In the vast majority of cases, double bonds cause kinks or bends in fatty acids, preventing them from lying flat. In fact, the more double bonds, the more bent the acids are. And that means they can't pile up or pack together like neatly stacked planks of wood. They are more fluid, like uncut logs flowing down a river.

It's for that reason that if a fat has mostly polyunsaturated fatty acids, like soybean and safflower oil, they won't pack together well and the oil is liquid at room temperature. And if a fat has mostly saturated fatty acids, they will not be bent and therefore will stack up against one another—which is why foods with a lot of saturated fat, like butter, are solid at room temperature. As you will see in chapter 5, saturated fats should be limited as much as possible. Poly- and monounsaturated fats should be used instead.

the typical American diet, which contains about 13 percent of calories as saturated fat, to a diet with only 7 percent of calories as saturated fat decreased their LDL-cholesterol by 10 percent. On average, however, research has shown that decreasing saturated fat intake by 5 percent of calories and replacing it with the same amount of polyunsaturated fat will reduce LDL-cholesterol levels by about 7 percent. That's still excellent. Overall, each 1 percent decrease in cholesterol levels has been associated with a 2 percent reduction in incidence of coronary heart disease.

Trans-*fatty acids*

A type of fat that is not saturated but which research has shown behaves similarly to saturated fat, or is perhaps slightly more harmful, is *trans* fat. Commonly referred to as *trans*-fatty acids, *trans* fat increases LDL-cholesterol levels. Unlike saturated fat, which also increases HDL-cholesterol levels, *trans* fat does not.

In practical terms, it is a moot point to debate which is worse in our diets because we consume relatively small amounts of *trans* fat compared with saturated fat. However, as with saturated fat, we would still benefit if we decreased intake. Indeed, in a Tufts research project, women who were fed diets that were relatively high in *trans* fat had almost 10 percent higher LDL-cholesterol levels than women whose diets contained low levels of *trans* fats.

While a small amount of *trans* fat occurs naturally in foods of animal origin, most of it comes from the hydrogenated vegetable oils in processed foods. The process of hydrogenation turns liquid vegetable oils into solids. Think of vegetable shortening and traditional stick margarine.

Now, you may think to yourself, "I don't cook with shortening or stick margarine, so I don't eat *trans*-fatty acids." Not true. There are probably still *trans*-fatty acids in your diet. Most of the *trans* fat we eat comes from foods like store-bought cakes, cookies, crackers, and other items. They also come from fried foods—either from your supermarket's frozen food section or fast-food chains and other restaurants.

Food manufacturers are currently in the process of adding to Nutrition Facts labels the amounts of *trans* fat in their products. The labeling changes will be complete by the end of 2005.

For your purposes, the labeling issue actually doesn't matter too much. When you get to the next chapter, you will see that most of the dietary recommendations we make include foods and food ingredients that contain little if any *trans*-fatty acids (and low amounts of saturated fat) to begin with.

Omega-3 Fatty Acids—A Special Kind of Polyunsaturated Fatty Acid

Polyunsaturated fatty acids, in place of saturated and *trans*-fatty acids, definitely help keep blood cholesterol as low as possible. But there are certain types of polyunsaturated fatty acids that outdo others when it comes to protecting the cardiovascular system. Called *omega-3 fatty acids,* they are

Is Olive Oil Better?

With the rise in popularity of the so-called Mediterranean diet, there came a rise in the popularity of olive oil, which is highest not in saturated or polyunsaturated fat but in monounsaturated fat. Fully 77 percent of the fatty acids in olive oil are monounsaturated, with 14 percent saturated and 9 percent polyunsaturated. A lot of people began thinking that if they just added olive oil to their diet, their blood cholesterol problems would be solved.

The same was thought of oils high in polyunsaturated fats in the early 1960s. There are stories of people who went to steak houses and followed up their sirloin entrées with a jigger of corn oil because it was high in polyunsaturated fat, as if one kind of fat could counteract or block the effects of another. It can't. It just adds calories, which leads to weight gain, and that generally leads to higher blood cholesterol levels. In other words, adding a particular kind of oil to the diet without subtracting another isn't simply useless—it's harmful.

In short, olive oil itself doesn't *lower* cholesterol levels, as some people believe. It lowers them only if you use it *in place of* saturated fat. And, as it turns out, research has shown that *other* vegetable oils, such as canola, which is lower in saturated fat than olive oil, is even more effective. So are soybean oil and corn oil, which are particularly high in polyunsaturated fat.

None of this is to say you shouldn't use olive oil. You should use it if you like the flavor. The two of us keep several types of oil in our houses: olive oil for salads; safflower or canola oil for cooking; and a little sesame oil for flavoring dishes with an Asian twist.

contained in fish and go under the names EPA (eicosapentaenoic acid) and DHA (docosahexaenoic acid).

EPA and DHA don't generally affect LDL-cholesterol levels. They appear to work in other ways. For instance, in one study recently published in the *American Journal of Clinical Nutrition* (called the Estrogen, Regression and

Atherosclerosis study, or ERA), it was demonstrated that women with diabetes who had already had a heart attack experienced a slower rate of atherosclerosis progression than similar women if they ate at least two fish meals a week or one fish meal that contained cold-water fish such as salmon or tuna. This was the first study in women to show a direct relationship between fish and slowed progression of atherosclerotic disease.

Other evidence in women indicates that those who eat *any* healthfully prepared fish, even as infrequently as a couple of times a month, have reduced rates of heart disease. Furthermore, if they suffer a coronary event, they are less likely to die.

Still other research suggests that the fat in fish makes blood platelets less "sticky" and therefore less likely to aggregate and form clots. It also appears to decrease the propensity of the heart to beat abnormally, a condition known as arrhythmia. Finally, fish promotes the relaxation of the lining of the blood vessels, which allows blood to flow more freely. In some people, it mildly decreases blood pressure.

Fatty, cold-water fish such as salmon seem to be more protective than white-flesh fish like cod. One reason, of course, is that fatty fish have more omega-3s. But also, white-fleshed fish is frequently battered and fried, which adds saturated (or sometimes *trans*) fat—and calories—that work to cancel out the effect of any omega-3s present. We will discuss some delicious ways to prepare fish healthfully in the next chapter.

Note that fish is not the only source of omega-3 fatty acids. They are also found in canola, soybean, and walnut oil, as well as in walnuts themselves. But the body has to convert the omega-3s in those foods to the heart-healthy EPA and DHA contained in fish. And it converts them very inefficiently, at a rate of 10 percent or less. Still, those oils (and nuts) are reasonable choices as part of a heart-healthy dietary pattern.

How Low Should Fat Go?
You may have heard that fat should make up no more than 30 percent of calories. But in the last couple of years, that guideline has been liberalized. It's okay for fat to comprise up to 35 percent of calories—as long as saturated fat and *trans*-fatty acids *combined* don't make up more than 10 percent of calories. We're not necessarily *advocating* a diet that gets 35 percent of calories from fat. A gram of fat contains more than twice as many calories as a

gram of carbohydrate or protein, so it can be easy to go overboard on calories on a somewhat high-fat diet. It's simply that if calories on a higher-fat diet can be kept low enough to keep you at a healthy weight, and it is the right kind of fat—polyunsaturated and monounsaturated and fat from fish—going up to 35 percent of calories as fat is not harmful.

At least as important, you should not go on a very low-fat diet, one in which less than 20 percent of calories come from fat. As fat intake goes down, carbohydrate intake goes up, and it has been well established that a very high-carbohydrate diet can raise triglyceride levels and keep down HDL-cholesterol. Consider that in one research trial, women and men whose diets were 29 percent fat had normal trigylceride levels averaging 115 and HDL-cholesterol concentrations averaging 42. But when fat was reduced to 15 percent of calories, triglycerides shot up to an average of 188, and HDL-cholesterol dropped to an average of 35.

Bottom line: Stick to a diet both moderate in fat and unprocessed carbohydrates—fruits, vegetables, legumes, and whole grains.

Counting Cholesterol

There has been a lot of confusion over cholesterol in the diet. Many people assume that the cholesterol in the foods you eat—eggs, meat, and full-fat dairy products like whole milk, butter, and ice cream—contributes directly to the amount of cholesterol in your bloodstream. Not true. Scientists have known for decades that how cholesterol gets into your blood is quite complex. In fact, saturated fat and *trans*-fatty acids are the major dietary determinants of cholesterol in your bloodstream, not the cholesterol you eat.

That said, the cholesterol in foods *can* increase blood cholesterol to some degree, more in some people than in others depending on genetics. Thus, if you're told you have elevated LDL-cholesterol, you should keep your dietary cholesterol at a maximum of 200 milligrams a day. Fortunately, if you're already following a diet that's low in saturated fat, that's easy to do. Most cholesterol-containing foods are also foods that contain a fair amount of saturated fat. (Eggs, which we'll discuss in the next chapter, are an exception.)

The Carbohydrate Connection

Forget everything you've heard about carbohydrates making you fat. They don't—unless you eat too many of them. But that's true of anything.

What's important to keep in mind about carbohydrates when it comes to heart disease is that certain carbohydrate-rich foods have clearly been associated with a decreased risk. The foods we're talking about are vegetables, fruits, and whole-grain items like whole-grain breads and cereals.

Why is not completely clear. As we said in chapter 3, it may have something to do with the fact that these foods all contain fiber, which is associated with better weight management and therefore with a reduced risk for heart problems. Fiber takes up a fair amount of room in the gut and apparently has the ability to help people feel sated even though it doesn't contain any calories.

Research has also shown that fiber helps keep down blood glucose and, to a small extent, helps lower blood cholesterol. In the ERA study, women who had suffered a heart attack and subsequently ate at least 3 grams of fiber from whole-grain foods every day, such as cereals and whole-wheat bread, experienced slower progression of atherosclerotic plaque afterward than women who consumed less fiber.

Some studies have even suggested that fiber decreases blood pressure. But it's also important to note that people who eat plenty of high-fiber foods have less room in their diets for high-calorie foods that can contribute to increased weight—and increased blood pressure.

Whatever the mechanism by which fiber works, hundreds, if not thousands, of studies have consistently shown a link between diets high in produce and low rates of chronic disease, including cardiovascular disease. It's the same for diets high in whole grains and produce.

The Protein Connection: Soy Story

While the kinds and amounts of carbohydrates and fats people eat can vary widely and have a significant effect on heart disease risk, Americans consume a pretty constant level of protein: about 15 percent of total calories (unless they follow one of the high-protein diets, which we don't recommend). While the type of fat the protein comes packaged with is important (there is saturated fat in beef, for instance, and largely unsaturated fat in fish), the protein itself doesn't have as much to do with heart health as is often thought—or bandied about in the press.

For a while it was believed that protein from soy-based foods such as tofu could significantly lower the chance of developing heart disease by lowering blood cholesterol, even to the point that claims for reduced heart-disease risk are now allowed on soy-containing foods. But while soy foods do make excellent protein substitutes for animal foods because they have virtually no saturated fat, the evidence that soy protein itself lowers cholesterol is much weaker than was originally thought. In one study conducted by Alice's group at the Cardiovascular Nutrition Laboratory, women and men who were fed a minimum of 50 grams of soy protein a day reduced their LDL-cholesterol by just 2 percent compared to those who were fed foods like steak and chicken instead. And 50 grams is a *lot*—the equivalent of almost 1½ pounds of tofu.

A similar but larger study conducted in Scandinavia recently corroborated this finding—and has also found that soy protein does not protect bone density (or cognitive function).

Specific Vitamins and Minerals

Fat, carbohydrates, and protein are known as the three macronutrients. They are the only nutrients that contribute calories to our diets (along with alcohol). There are also the micronutrients—vitamins and minerals—and emerging research has turned up some intriguing information on whether some of them can help stave off heart disease. In some cases, the findings have been promising. In others, the evidence of benefit has not been as strong as researchers originally hoped. In still other cases, the jury remains out. Whatever the evidence, it's important always to bear in mind that it's the dietary *pattern* that counts, not any particular nutrient in isolation. But it's good to know which single nutrients might be having an effect because it allows that pattern to be tailored to the best possible advantage.

B Vitamins

People who follow diets high in the B vitamins folate, B_6, and B_{12} have relatively low levels in the blood of homocysteine, a substance implicated in heart disease risk that we discussed in chapter 2. While the research is ongoing and we don't yet know whether reducing homocysteine levels by eating more foods with B vitamins actually reduces heart disease risk (we've gotten from point X to point Y but not from point Y to point Z), these vitamins are found in foods that belong in a heart-healthy eating pattern anyway. Folate, for instance, is contained in legumes such as kidney beans, chickpeas, and lentils, along with green leafy vegetables and orange juice. And since 1998, it must be added to refined-grain products, including breads, pasta, and white rice (which is why it's okay for *some* of your starch to be refined rather than whole). Vitamin B$_6$ is plentiful in vegetables as well as in fruits and can also be found in seafood, poultry, and beef. And B$_{12}$ is in all foods of animal origin. Thus, if you're eating right, B vitamins are keeping down homocysteine automatically, which is a can't-hurt, might-help part of the bargain.

Vitamin K

Found in highest concentrations in green leafy vegetables, vitamin K is now thought to possibly contribute to heart health in ways previously unidentified. Researchers in the Vitamin K Laboratory at Tufts are currently investigating whether it can help slow hardening of the arteries. There's already test tube and animal research that suggests as much. To test it in humans, investigators are giving more than 450 people either 500 micrograms of vitamin K every day or a placebo, or dummy pill. They will then look at their degree of vascular calcification down the line.

Currently, Americans consume an average of about 120 micrograms of vitamin K daily. But it's easy to get more. A half cup of cooked spinach contains 360 micrograms; a half cup of brussels sprouts (which amounts to just four sprouts), 235 micrograms; and a half cup of cooked collard greens, 400 micrograms. Even if vitamin K doesn't ultimately prove to protect against heart disease, eating more of these green vegetables is consistent with eating heart-healthy in general.

Calcium

When it comes to heart disease, calcium falls into the same category as vitamin K. The research suggests but doesn't prove that this nutrient may have something to do with reduced risk. Specifically, there's a body of research that suggests calcium might help regulate blood pressure, especially when consumed as part of a diet high in fruits and vegetables. Some research, albeit extremely thin, even suggests it may be associated with helping to keep down blood cholesterol.

The good news here: You don't need to wait for definitive results before you incorporate more calcium in your diet. *All* women should eat at least two, preferably three, servings of high-calcium foods every day anyway, to avoid osteoporosis. Skim and 1 percent milk, low- and nonfat yogurt, canned salmon or sardines with the bones, many brands of tofu and soy milk (check Nutrition Fact labels), an ounce to an ounce and a half of hard cheese, calcium-fortified juices and cereals—all of these fill the bill as high-calcium choices. Smaller but still significant amounts of calcium can be found in broccoli, oranges, figs, and other plant-based foods.

Vitamin E
Hopes were originally very high for the role of vitamin E supplements in preventing heart disease, so much so that many physicians still recommend it to their patients. But while observations of large populations suggested a protective effect from vitamin E supplements, numerous carefully controlled studies in which some people were given vitamin E pills and others a placebo have not panned out. The E takers were no more protected from future heart attacks and other cardiovascular events than the non–E takers. (As far as vitamin E and immune function along with protection against cancer, the jury is still out, despite claims in ads and the popular press.)

Potassium
The National Academy of Sciences recommends that people consume 4,700 milligrams of potassium daily. That's the amount deemed necessary for helping to stave off high blood pressure. Potassium is found mostly in fruits and vegetables (see page 67). Currently, Americans, including women, average only about 2,300 milligrams of potassium a day.

To raise it high enough, it would be necessary to double produce consumption from the current national average of four to five servings a day to eight to ten servings daily.

That's exactly what the DASH diet suggests. DASH is an acronym for Dietary Approaches to Stop Hypertension, an eating plan that so successfully lowered blood pressure in research studies that it has been endorsed by the National Heart, Lung, and Blood Institute.

The Details Come Together in the DASH Diet
In 1997 scientists from six major medical centers around the country first tested the DASH diet. In that trial, participants were provided with a diet

aining eight to ten daily servings of fruits and vegetables, two to three ings of low-fat dairy foods, and a couple of small portions of meat, chicken, or fish—all of which ensured that they were consuming plenty of potassium, calcium, B vitamins, and other nutrients that research has found look promising for preventing heart disease in general. The upshot: the DASH diet was significantly more effective at lowering blood pressure than the typical American diet that is low in produce as well as high-calcium dairy items. In a follow-up study in 2000, the researchers went a step further, putting people on essentially the same DASH diet but manipulating certain foods so that the study participants were at one of three sodium levels: 3,300 milligrams a day (about as much as many women eat); 2,400 milligrams a day (less than many women consume); or 1,500 milligrams a day (less than virtually anyone in this country eats). It turned out that the lower the sodium level, the more blood pressure dropped—even for people whose blood pressure started out in the normal or high-normal ranges. That's important because generally speaking, the lower your blood pressure, the lower your risk for stroke and heart disease.

With some tweaking to reflect findings about heart disease prevention that have come out since the DASH diet was tested, the recommendations of our dietary plan in the next chapter largely coincide with the recommendations of DASH: plenty of produce and low-fat dairy products and modest portions of meat with little in the way of sweets and salty snacks. And because our plan is based largely on whole foods that have not gone through a lot of processing, it's naturally low in sodium.

THE EXERCISE UNDERPINNINGS

Diet is *half* of what you need to focus on, lifestyle-wise, to protect your heart. The other half is physical activity. Researchers are coming to understand, in fact, that the two together are absolutely vital for the best heart health possible. Yes, you have to eat right to treat your arteries and heart well. But if you don't challenge your body by working it through exercise, your heart muscle and the rest of your cardiovascular system will not work at their best levels. All the good eating in the world, while crucial in its own right, isn't enough to counteract a sedentary lifestyle.

Aerobics

In 1968, Dr. Kenneth Cooper published a book called *Aerobics,* both coining a new term and marking the beginning of a fitness revolution. Aerobics— brisk walking, running, swimming, biking, and other activities during which the body is in continuous motion—challenges your heart, lungs, and entire vascular system to work harder and thereby makes them stronger and more efficient at their jobs. People who participate regularly in aerobics have lower heart rates, which, as you'll recall from chapter 2, means they need fewer beats per minute to pump oxygen- and nutrient-rich blood from the heart to the rest of the body.

But it wasn't until ten years after Dr. Cooper's book came out—1978— that aerobics was put on the scientific map as a significant contributor to reduced risk of heart disease. That year, a researcher from Stanford University named Ralph Paffenbarger, M.D., published a remarkable study in the *Journal of Epidemiology.* He and his colleagues had studied almost 17,000 Harvard alumni (all men) ages 35 to 74. All had entered Harvard sometime between 1916 and 1950.

Using answers to questionnaires, Dr. Paffenbarger and his colleagues learned that more than 500 of the men had already had a heart attack. They also learned how many stairs the men climbed and blocks they walked daily as well as to what degree they participated in strenuous sports. In other words, they got a handle on the men's current degree of aerobic activity. What the researchers found was that the men who burned at least 2,000 calories a week in aerobic activities were 64 percent less likely to have been one of the heart attack sufferers. They also found—and this is crucial—that the men's current aerobic habits were much more predictive of their heart health than their physical activity patterns while they were in college. Having been athletic decades before doesn't offset a sedentary lifestyle now. Or, put more positively, becoming aerobically active in middle or old age has a lot more bearing on your heart health than having been sedentary in your twenties. Age matters less; it's what you do today that counts.

But Do the Findings Apply Directly to Women?

At around the same time that West Coast researchers at Stanford were finding that exercise protects men's hearts, East Coast investigators at Harvard were gearing up to start the long-running Nurses' Health Study, which began in the late 1970s with almost 122,000 female nurses from around the country who were between 30 and 55. The study was originally set up to look at the health effects of the birth control pill. But the scientists quickly realized they were working with an enormously rich resource for studying issues in women that hadn't yet been systematically studied—diet, exercise, body weight, and smoking, and the effect of those lifestyle factors on disease, health, and longevity. Here are some of the findings, reported intermittently over the years, as the study went (and continues to go) forward:

- Women who walk at a brisk pace for at least three hours a week reduce their risk for heart attacks and other coronary events by 35 percent compared to women who walk only infrequently. The same holds true for reducing their risk for diabetes.
- Women who engage in the most physical activity each week— equivalent to about a half hour a day of very brisk walking—are at a 34 percent decreased risk of suffering a stroke compared to those who exercise the least.
- Physical activity helps to protect women from heart disease even if they are at high risk because they are overweight or they smoke. They are not as well protected as exercisers who are of normal weight and don't smoke, but they are significantly more protected than sedentary overweight women and smokers.

The Nurses' Health Study isn't the only one that links women's cardiovascular health to physical activity. The Cooper Institute for Aerobics Research in Dallas now has data on more than 40,000 women and men combined. The first, and most classic, research paper on some of them appeared in 1989 in the *Journal of the American Medical Association*. In an eight-year study that included more than 3,000 women and 10,000 men, it was found that those in the bottom 20 percent of fitness ranking were 65 percent more likely to die from heart attacks and strokes (and diabetes and cancer!) than the 20 percent of people in the top fitness ranking, as measured by treadmill test performance.

Johns Hopkins Medical Institutions researcher Samia Mora, M.D., obtained corroborating findings in her research just a couple of years ago. Almost 3,000 women ages 30 to 80 with no symptoms indicative of a bad heart underwent treadmill tests in the 1970s. They were observed for exercise capacity—how intensely they could go at it on a treadmill—and also for the amount of time it took for their heartbeats to return to normal after they stopped exercising. Twenty years later, those who had not been able to work up to an intensity equivalent to walking about five miles an hour (which is a very brisk pace) and whose heart rates did not "recover" by declining toward resting rate by at least 55 beats per minute were three and a half times more likely than those with better numbers to have died of heart disease—or *any* other cause. **Exercise ability was so strongly linked with the risk of death that even a sedentary woman who had desirable blood cholesterol levels, didn't smoke, and didn't have high blood pressure was at six times the risk of dying from heart disease as a very active woman with the same desirable cholesterol and blood pressure.**

The upside here: Exercise capacity, or fitness, can be improved significantly even with moderate physical activity in just a matter of months. It goes back to the fact that even if you've been inactive your whole life, you can dramatically lower your risk of dying prematurely simply by walking briskly or engaging in other aerobic activities on a regular basis *now*. You'll lower your blood pressure (as dozens of clinical trials have shown) and blood cholesterol (as dozens of other trials have shown), not to mention help control your weight, improve your overall function and quality of life, and get better-quality sleep.

No wonder the Surgeon General, the Dietary Guidelines for Americans, and the American Heart Association all say that people should set a goal of at least 30 minutes of moderate-intensity physical activity (15 to 20 minutes per mile) on most (preferably all) days of the week. Even more cardiovascular gains will be accrued by exercising *vigorously* for 20 to 40 minutes three to five days per week—to the point where you break a sweat.

Unfortunately, as awareness about the benefits of aerobic activity has increased, actual participation in aerobics has leveled off after increasing through the sixties, seventies, and eighties. Only 27 percent of Americans get enough exercise to benefit them, and 38 percent of American women are not active at all.

Aerobic Exercise Starts Working *Immediately*

Of course, the more frequently you exercise, the greater the benefits to your heart. But some effects are immediate. Consider
that triglycerides are reduced right away by vigorous exercise and that
the effects last up to seventy-two hours. Similarly, exercise causes
transient upticks in HDL-cholesterol, reduces blood pressure for up
to twelve hours, and improves glucose uptake by the cells.

And preliminary evidence suggests that just a single bout of exercise helps your heart rate become more variable. Why would you
want your heart rate to become more variable?

The reason, new research suggests, is that women who have a very
stable, nonvarying resting heart rate (*beat, beat, beat*) are at greater
risk for cardiac events—and death—than women whose resting heart
rate keeps shifting (*beat, beat, beatbeat, beat*). A steady, unchanging
heart rate means your heart is not able to respond to tiny fluctuations
in body processes. A heart that can adapt to and accommodate the
body's subtle changes in needs moment to moment can help keep
things more fine-tuned.

Sedentary women who are older are particularly apt to have compromised heart rate variability; over time, there is a decline in the ability
of the heart to react moment by moment to changes in the need for
blood flow and oxygen in the rest of the body. But, and this is a big
but, when a team of scientists in France set out to evaluate the impact
that exercise has on heart rate variability in adults with an average age
of 75, they found that those who were regularly active had significantly higher heart rate variability than their more unfit counterparts. The bottom line: With exercise you can become young at heart,
literally, improving the heart muscle's ability to adapt quickly and
thereby help reduce the risk of a heart attack, stroke, or other cardiovascular calamity.

Strength Training

When you think about exercising for heart health, chances are you think about aerobic activities like walking and bicycling, which makes sense, since they directly affect heart and lung capacity. But more and more research is bringing to light the fact that strength training improves heart health, too.

The most obvious reason is that strength training improves aerobic capabilities. Former Tufts colleagues of ours proved this point when they studied patients in a local cardiac rehabilitation program. All the patients participated in walking several times weekly, but only half strength-trained three times a week. After twenty-one weeks, the aerobic gains made by the strength trainers were 18 percent greater. Why? When you increase the strength of your muscles, including your leg muscles, through strength training, walking becomes easier. That, in turn, lets you walk faster and farther, which gives the heart and lungs a better workout.

But strength training does more than allow for better aerobic training. Studies have also shown that people who lift weights regularly have lower blood pressure. One study was conducted here at Tufts by Carmen Castaneda, M.D., a close colleague of Miriam's. After sixteen weeks, women and men who had been enrolled in a strength-training program experienced significant reductions in blood pressure. They also lost fat around the abdomen, which presents more of a heart disease risk than fat on the hips, thighs, and buttocks.

Perhaps most important, the participants, all of whom had diabetes, experienced significant improvements in blood sugar—to the point that most of them were able to reduce their diabetes medication. That's no small achievement since, as we've noted, diabetes itself greatly increases the risk for heart disease.

It has been common knowledge for many years that exercise helps control diabetes. But the research has generally looked at aerobic exercise. Now we know that strength training is a critical element in the arsenal of lifestyle approaches to help women control this disease. (The information comes none too soon. Diabetes is on the rise in the United States, with a 700 percent increase since 1960. An estimated 16 million Americans have it, and another 17 million are pre-diabetic. And the age at which people are getting it, because of increasing weight coupled with increasing physical inactivity, is getting younger and younger. It's no longer just a condition of middle and old age.)

As for strength training's ability to reduce the rate of heart disease directly, results from trials on women are still pending. But in a Harvard study of more than 40,000 men, it was found that those who strength-trained more than thirty minutes a week had a reduction in cardiovascular risk of about 30 percent. We suspect the same will be found true in women.

Strength training does not take as much time as aerobics. Twice a week, thirty to forty minutes per session, will suffice.

DIET AND EXERCISE: THE WHOLE PACKAGE

The best part about the heart-healthy benefits of the right dietary patterns and the right kinds of exercise is that they are all in your hands. That is, research has proven unequivocally that whether or not you substantially decrease your risk for heart disease is very much up to you. You're not "stuck" with a particular heart disease risk because of your genes or your family history or because "things are the way they are." Indeed, the scientific evidence from the 100,000-plus women in the Nurses' Health Study suggests that women who eat a healthful diet and exercise regularly (and don't smoke and maintain a desirable body weight) can enjoy up to an 84 percent reduction in the risk of cardiovascular death.

Yet only 3 percent of the women studied were in that heart-healthy lifestyle category. In fact, as we alluded to earlier, the American lifestyle has become so far removed from what is good for us that deaths from poor diet and inactivity will soon overtake deaths from smoking.

We hope to change those numbers dramatically. In the next section, we give clear, detailed instructions for how to translate the dietary and exercise research into a lifestyle you can live with—and enjoy! You'll see that eating well and incorporating more physical activity into your days will feel so good, you'll never want to return to your old habits.

PART 2

The Strong Women, Strong Hearts Program

CHAPTER 5

Don't Think Diet— Think Food Patterns

◆

I had kind of let everything go. Before menopause, my cholesterol used to be really low. After, it was much higher. At the same time, I was eating all the bad stuff—too many desserts, too much sugar, too many cookies. I needed to get back on the bandwagon and start eating real food. I started by eating more fruits and vegetables, drinking mostly water if I was thirsty. Now I eat a lot of salads. I put in currants or pine nuts or sunflower seeds, avocado, tomato, scallions, cucumber. Maybe a little bit of crumbled feta cheese. And I dress it with olive oil, a little balsamic vinegar, garlic, and a splash of lemon juice. I realized I wasn't going to stick with it if it was too boring. I didn't want to eat just plain vegetables. I wanted it interesting. It had to taste good, and I had to be able to look forward to it.

—WENDY

Conjure up the word "diet," and the words "restrictive," "punishing," "boring," and "lacking flavor" won't be far behind. That's because so often, when health professionals as well as the media talk about diet, they talk about things you shouldn't eat, foods you can no longer enjoy. It's as though the whole world has become the proverbial finger-wagging lady with a hair net in the school cafeteria, the one who has nothing tasty to offer and heaps limp, overcooked green beans onto your plate with a scowl. The food-can't-taste-good notion is especially deep-rooted when it comes to diets for preventing disease. After all, if you want to keep your heart healthy into old age and also substantially stunt unhealthful rises in blood pressure, there has to be an onerous tradeoff, right? Stay away from fat, stay away from meat, watch this, watch that.

Well, guess what? Eating for heart health happens to be delicious, as we both know firsthand and will show you with menu ideas and recipe suggestions. Heart-healthy eating is taste, it's texture, it's color—it's enjoyment. As well it must be. Like Wendy says, if you don't like what you eat, your eating plan will backfire because it will not become your default mode—what you automatically do instead of what you *have* to do. Sure, you may experience an episodic burst of enthusiasm for a diet you don't like because you feel motivated, initially, to take care of your health. But if you have to give up too much in the way of gustatory satisfaction or it becomes too cumbersome to adhere to in your everyday life, that enthusiasm is going to wane—fast— and you'll be back where you started.

More good news about a heart-healthy diet: On top of its being something you'll be *glad* to incorporate into your lifestyle, following it will protect not just your heart health but also your health in general. That's right. Eating heart healthfully will decrease your risk for developing diabetes, hypertension, some cancers, osteoporosis, and a host of other ills—for *anyone.* If you're raising children or sharing your life with a significant other, you will be imprinting important health-promoting behaviors onto the lifestyle template of those you love.

YOU DON'T NEED A DEGREE IN SCIENCE TO DO THIS

In the previous chapter, we went through a good deal of research to show you the bases of our recommendations. But you don't need to be a scientific investigator to eat right, constantly counting milligrams or calculating percentages. Putting our nutrition program into practice is deceptively *un*complicated. It will work no matter what your eating style—meat eater, vegetarian, or somewhere in between. That's because it is really a dietary *pattern* rather than prescriptions for or against particular foods and so can be adapted to accommodate almost any dietary preferences or restrictions. It simply involves keeping the emphasis on the whole foods available on the perimeter of the

Is There Such a Thing as a
Cholesterol-Lowering Food?

Are there really foods that can legitimately be called *cholesterol low-erers*? For instance, one often hears that oatmeal is a cholesterol-lowering food.

We don't believe it's a good idea to think of individual foods that way. Foods don't work in isolation. They work in concert with all the other foods you eat. That is, you can't eat a bowl of oatmeal and follow it up with a hot fudge sundae and expect to lower your blood cholesterol. A food can only work as well as the whole nutrition plan it's fit into.

Thus, when you read or hear that a single food is good for the heart, the questions you have to ask yourself are: What am I going to give up if I add in the new food? Is it high in saturated fat or *trans*-fatty acids? Low in fiber? Will I be forgoing as many calories as I'm going to be consuming with the new item? If you decide the food is a good choice for you, then by all means include it in your heart-healthy eating plan—if you happen to like it.

Keep in mind that if you're already eating a healthy pattern of foods that don't contain too many calories and have plenty of fiber and other healthful components, making room for one particular food isn't going to make all that much difference. And if you're not eating well to begin with, adding that food won't overcome the overall shortcomings, either. It takes more than one food to change your food-eating pattern.

supermarket (the produce and dairy aisles, for instance) rather than on the boxed, bagged, canned, and other packaged goods lining all the center aisles. Those choices often contain too little fiber, too many refined carbohydrates that lack certain nutrients, and frequently too much in the way of sugar, saturated and *trans* fats, and salt. Stick to whole and minimally processed foods, and sooner than you think, they will become the choices you *want*, not the way you have to eat.

Wendy puts it this way: "I got to a point where I wanted to eat as 'real' as I could, instead of eating quick, fast junk. I soon found I wasn't eating things from bottles, jars, and boxes. I literally had less trash to put out. The good stuff isn't just going to appear in your refrigerator. You have to watch what you put there; you have to make the shift. But once you start to do it, it's just like junk food—it becomes a habit."

That doesn't mean you can never have some potato chips or boxed convenience food ever again. *Any* food can fit into a heart-healthy diet, at least once in a while. It just means that most of your choices will have undergone little to no tampering at a food-processing plant.

To keep the focus on the delicious, nutrient-dense foods that will form the centerpiece of your heart-healthy eating plan, keep in mind this HEART acronym:

H eap on the vegetables and fruits.
E mphasize the right fats.
A ccentuate whole grains.
R evere low- and nonfat dairy foods.
T arget heart-healthy proteins.

Now we'll take a closer look at each of these points.

Heap on the Vegetables and Fruits

GOAL: seven to nine servings daily

SERVING SIZE: 1 cup raw leafy vegetables, such as lettuce or spinach
                1 cup raw vegetables, cut up
                ½ cup cooked vegetables
                ¾ cup vegetable juice
                1 medium fruit, such as an apple, pear, or orange
                1 cup raw fruit (sliced or chopped)
                1 cup berries, grapes, or other small fruit
                ½ cup cooked, frozen, or canned (in its own juice) fruit
                ¼ cup dried fruit
                ¾ cup 100% fruit juice

Vegetable and Fruit Powerhouses

Fiber-Rich

All vegetables and fruits (but not juices) are good sources of fiber. Below are some particularly high-fiber choices. The Daily Value for fiber is 25 grams. (Remember, some of your fiber will also come from whole grains and beans.)

	Grams of fiber
1 cup of raspberries	8
1 pear	4
1 cup blueberries	4
1 apple	4
½ cup cooked peas	4
½ cup cooked brussels sprouts	3
1 orange	3
½ cup cooked spinach	3
1 banana	3
1 small baked potato with skin	3

Plenty of Potassium

The recommendation for potassium is 4,700 milligrams. (Currently, Americans average about 2,500 milligrams.) Following are some particularly potassium-rich vegetables and fruits. (Other nutritious foods are good sources of potassium, too. A cup of plain yogurt has 531 milligrams; 3 ounces of cooked halibut or tuna steak, almost 500 milligrams.)

	Milligrams of potassium
1 small baked potato with skin	593
1 cup cantaloupe chunks	494
1 baked sweet potato with skin	493
1 banana	467
½ cup cooked winter squash	448
½ cup cooked spinach	420
¾ cup orange juice	355

If we were designing our own food guide pyramid, vegetables and fruits, rather than grains, would form the base. What makes us feel so strongly here is the *consistency* with which studies have shown that diets rich in vegetables and fruits are associated with a decreased risk for developing heart disease and stroke.

How many servings of produce should you be eating a day? The standard advice is at least five, but we believe there is good reason to eat more on the order of seven to nine. At the very least, that much will get you closer to the 25 grams of fiber that adults should eat daily. And produce is low in calories compared to many other types of foods. Therefore, if it becomes a mainstay in your diet, you have a better shot at successful weight management by virtue of its replacing other, higher-calorie options. Produce is also high in potassium and generally very low in sodium, both of which are associated with decreased blood pressure.

Note that we say "vegetables and fruits," not "fruits and vegetables." This is not by chance. Fruits are great for you, but vegetables, in particular, tend to be nutrient-rich and are hard to overdo because they're relatively low in calories. We recommend at least four to five servings of vegetables daily and two to four of fruit, preferably not in the form of juice.

If you really love ¾ cup of orange or grapefruit juice in the morning and you don't have a weight problem, fine. But whole fruit, unlike juice, offers fiber. And it tends to be more filling. An orange will stave off mid-morning hunger much better than a glass of orange juice. (We'll explain further in chapter 7.)

Incorporating more produce into your diet is not hard *at all,* especially when you consider that frozen is just as nutritious as fresh and is easy to keep in the house. If you buy it in bags rather than boxes, you can always take from the freezer as much or as little as you like. Tips for increasing vegetables and fruits throughout the day:

- Heat some frozen spinach, broccoli, or sliced brussels sprouts in the microwave or on the stove to have with dinner or to top a toasted whole-wheat English muffin with melted cheese for lunch.
- Make a chicken salad that's half chopped celery and shredded carrots and half chicken.
- Into either your own homemade tomato sauce or into prepared sauce, toss finely chopped or grated vegetables. This is great for

Potatoes: A Vegetable or a Starch?

Potatoes have been much maligned in recent years as bad "carbs" that will send your blood sugar soaring and make you fat. Don't be too quick to judge. Potatoes are decent vegetables that have been unfairly criticized. Their skin is a good source of fiber, and the fleshy part contains lots of potassium and a reasonable amount of vitamin C, along with other nutrients.

Potatoes *are* starchier than other vegetables, meaning they do have a lot of carbohydrates, similar to grains. In fact, culturally and culinarily, they are generally used as a starch rather than as a vegetable per se. And like starches, they also contain more calories than other vegetables ounce for ounce. For example, there are 26 calories in an ounce of baked potato, compared with only 7 in an ounce of cooked broccoli. That totals 128 calories for a smallish potato, and much more if potatoes are turned into fries—the way most potatoes are consumed in the United States. Along with calories, fries usually contain *trans*-fatty acids because of the fat they are fried in.

Even if you eat a potato baked rather than fried, adding a lot of butter and sour cream cuts into its healthfulness by making it much more caloric—and not the best choice for your heart because those toppings are extremely high in saturated fat.

For that reason, we suggest that you use small baked potatoes (preferably with the skin), or split a larger one between two people, topping it with a little low-fat sour cream, or perhaps low-fat yogurt mixed with chives. And think of potatoes as a grain rather than a vegetable. That is, they're not "instead of" broccoli; they're instead of bread, rice, or pasta.

Keep in mind, too, that potatoes are only one tasty side-dish starch. There are lots of whole-grain starches that are delicious but that people make too little use of, as you'll see on page 72, in "Accentuate Whole Grains."

family members who aren't big on produce because it doesn't change the taste much.

- Consider adding vegetables where they may not have been before. For example, if preparing lasagna, mix thawed chopped spinach with the ricotta cheese. Or slice an eggplant into ¼-inch-thick slices, dribble on vegetable oil, bake at 400°F until soft, and use as its own lasagna layer.
- Keep frozen berries on hand to top yogurt or ice cream. Just thaw them in the microwave before using.
- Toss a handful of dried cranberries into a green salad with feta cheese and vinaigrette.
- Make one of Miriam's one-minute fruit smoothies for an afternoon snack: Throw into the blender a cup of nonfat yogurt, a half cup of frozen berries or other frozen fruit of your choice, and a splash of blueberry or grape juice; blend for 30 seconds, and presto.

We are fortunate that more and more fruits are available at reasonable prices year-round. Always keep a bowl of fruit within easy reach. For fruit that ripens quickly, such as peaches and nectarines, put out only a few at a time. Better to have a small bowl with a limited number of fruits that look good in order to make them more appealing. If you do this, fruit will become the default snack.

It's that way with produce in general. Availability translates into consumption. If you always have fresh, frozen, or canned on hand, you'll eat it (and may even eat less of other foods that aren't so heart-healthy).

Emphasize the Right Fats

Given the typical American diet, the first order of the day is to reduce consumption of heart-unhealthy fats. That includes the saturated fat in beef, poultry, and other meat as well as full-fat dairy foods, and the *trans*-fatty acids in commercially fried and baked foods and other items, including the legions of packaged foods that run the gamut from cookies, cakes, and crackers to microwavable popcorn and frozen entrées.

But you can also improve your diet by choosing the fats, or oils, most conducive to heart health. As we said before, a low-fat diet is no longer considered the right way to go. It's a *moderate*-fat diet, as long as you have the right fats.

The omega-3 fatty acids in fish are a great help, of course.

When it comes to cooking, the best bets are most vegetable oils. These include canola, safflower, sunflower, corn, olive, and soybean oil. Canola is the lowest in saturated fat of all cooking oils, with all the others close behind. When we say "vegetable oil," we are always referring to one of these, any of which is heart-healthy. We think it's best to keep a few different types in the house for particular uses, such as sautéeing vegetables, dressing salads, and so on.

Nutrition researchers as well as public health experts used to make a big distinction between oils high in monounsaturated fatty acids, such as olive

Are Nuts Especially Heart Healthy?

You may have heard a lot about nuts recently. There's even a health claim about them, approved by the FDA, saying they might help reduce the risk for heart disease: "Scientific evidence suggests but does not prove that eating 1.5 ounces per day of most nuts as part of a diet low in saturated fat and cholesterol may reduce the risk of heart disease." It's true that nuts, like other plant-based foods, are low in saturated fat, devoid of cholesterol, and high in unsaturated fats. But will increasing your consumption of nuts actually decrease your risk of developing cardiovascular disease? It depends. If you replace your mid-afternoon snack of a candy bar with an equivalent number of calories from nuts (there are 160 to 180 in an ounce), you will be decreasing your intake of saturated fat and *trans*-fatty acids, and that's all to the good. But switching from a plain chocolate bar to one with almonds will not likely confer any benefit. And adding nuts without subtracting something else most certainly will not be beneficial, since increased calories will lead to weight gain.

The bottom line: If you enjoy nuts in salads or on yogurt, or plain as a snack, by all means eat them. But when you add nuts to your diet, something else has to come out. Preferably the food you will be eating less of is high in *trans* or saturated fatty acids.

and canola oil, and those high in polyunsaturated fatty acids, such as safflower, sunflower, and corn oil. It was thought olive oil was particularly beneficial for reducing heart disease risk. However, the scientific evidence no
longer supports that line of thinking. The aim is simply to shoot for more
unsaturated fat and less saturated and *trans* fats. That's the best way of keeping down cholesterol levels.

When it comes to solid rather than liquid fats, go with soft (tub or
squeezable) margarine over butter or stick margarine (unless the label says
it's *trans* fat–free). Or use nonbutter blends with little to no saturated fat or
trans-fatty acids per serving. Despite the flak over margarine several years
ago when it was discovered that the *trans*-fatty acids contained in traditional
stick margarine raise LDL-cholesterol as much as the saturated fat found in
butter, there's not much difference between the two. You should limit both.
Generally speaking, the softer or more liquid the margarine, the less saturated *and trans* fats it has than other spreads.

Accentuate Whole Grains

GOAL: Four to nine servings daily (at least half from whole grain)

SERVING SIZE: 1 (1-oz.) slice bread

½ cup rice, pasta, or other cooked grain

½ cup cooked oatmeal

1 serving breakfast cereal (refer to label for serving size)

½ English muffin

½ (2-oz.) bagel

No food component has taken as much of a beating in the public consciousness in the last five years as carbohydrates—the major components of grains.
They have been branded *the* villain of all weight-control efforts.

Well, we have some news for you. It's not true. Carbohydrates are GOOD
FOR YOU! Granted, a recent report from the Centers for Disease Control
and Prevention points to carbohydrate-rich foods as the ones that have
added most of the 300-plus calories daily to the average woman's diet over
the last thirty years. But the bulk of those calories come from *refined* carbohydrates, such as the sugar (high fructose corn syrup) in soda pop or

desserts, and the white flour used to make pizza dough and most pasta, salty snacks like pretzels, and the refined flour in cakes, cookies, and the like. That is, the problem is not with carbohydrate-rich grains. It's with the particular forms of grains too many of us are eating too much of.

The grains that are heart-healthy are *whole* grains—whole-grain breads and cereals, brown rice, and whole-wheat pasta. Unlike refined grains, they contain fiber plus a host of nutrients and healthful plant chemicals that are eliminated when grains go through the refining process. No wonder whole grains are the ones that research has shown are associated with decreased heart disease risk in women.

The problem is that whole-grain foods are hard to come by. Only 5 percent of the packaged grain-based products you'll find in the supermarket are whole grain. And it's not easy to tell which ones they are. Terms such as "multi-grain," "seven-grain," and "unbleached flour" on food labels for breads, muffins, waffles, and the like all sound as though the product is whole grain. But they don't mean a thing as far as whether a grain is truly whole or not. Even "whole wheat" bagels sold at one popular doughnut/ bagel chain are not whole wheat. You have to look past the name on the front of the package to the fine print on the ingredients list. If the word "whole" is part of the first ingredient listed, the food contains whole grain. If not, pass it up. If the label says "100% whole grain" or "whole wheat," so much the better. Pretty much the only exceptions in packaged foods are oats and rice. Oats are automatically a whole grain. They are not stripped of their whole-grain components, even if the word "whole" does not appear on the packaging. And if the rice is *brown* rice, the whole rice grain is in the package. It hasn't gone through refining.

Fortunately, there are other whole-grain options besides breads, cereals, rice, and related products. One is popcorn. Yes, popcorn; corn is a whole grain. Just make sure it's air-popped rather than made with butter or partially hydrogenated fat (*trans*-fatty acids).

There are also whole grains that you can cook up as starches either for side dishes or for breakfast. For instance, wheatberries are a whole grain that Miriam turns into one of her favorite morning meals (see recipe at the end of this chapter). There's also bulgur, buckwheat groats (kasha), barley, millet, spelt, faro, and quinoa (pronounced KEEN-wah). These grains can be served

Salt Shakedown

The amount of salt or, more specifically, sodium in your diet is related to your blood pressure. The more salt you consume each day, the higher your blood pressure is going to be. That said, we all differ in our response to salt; some women's blood pressure is going to drop much more than others' in response to a decline in salt consumption. Still, eating less salt is certainly not harmful and most likely will be beneficial, especially as you age. Most people become more "salt sensitive" as they get older, with a bigger change in blood pressure depending on the amount of salt they eat.

What's the best way to reduce your salt intake? The vast majority of the salt we eat, as much as 80 percent, comes from prepared foods. If you follow our advice in this chapter and eat a diet that is predominantly composed of unprocessed foods, you will have more control of your salt intake. There are also some simple rules to follow:

- Don't add salt to your food until you taste it to make certain it really needs it.
- Don't put a saltshaker on the table.
- Don't use salt directly out of the package you buy it in, even for cooking. Transfer some to a shaker so that it is easier to control the amount you add to the food you are preparing.
- If you can see grains of salt on a product, look for one with less.

Many products are now available in "reduced salt" or "low-sodium" versions. Try them, especially if you are using them for cooking. You can always add salt, whereas you can't take it out.

Keep in mind that we can "unlearn" our taste for salt. Our love of sugar is inborn. With salt, within months of cutting back, what was once "salty enough" will become "too salty." Try it and see.

plain and can take the place of brown rice or pasta. Just check the package or a cookbook for preparation instructions.

Whole grains are always available in natural foods markets but can also be found in many traditional supermarkets, either with the regular items, such as brown rice and whole-wheat pasta, or in the "natural foods" section.

We are not saying that every single carbohydrate-rich food you eat has to be a whole grain. But the more, the better—*at least half.* Bear in mind that a lot of grain-based foods contain several servings at once. A 5-ounce bagel from a coffee shop equals five servings from the grains group, not one. Two cups of pasta at an Italian restaurant count as four servings of grains, since a single serving is a half cup. Granted, if that is the centerpiece of the meal, it might be perfectly appropriate to eat several servings at once. What is important is to be aware of it and factor it into your daily food pattern.

Revere Low- and Nonfat Dairy Foods

GOAL: two to three servings daily

SERVING SIZE: 1 cup nonfat or 1% milk

1 cup low- or nonfat yogurt

1 ounce hard cheese (cheddar, Swiss, etc.)

1½ ounces reduced-fat hard cheese

½ cup part-skim ricotta cheese

½ cup nonfat or 1% fat cottage cheese

As every woman knows, dairy products are associated with stronger bones and may keep down blood pressure. All are excellent sources of protein as well as outstanding sources of calcium and other nutrients. It is important to choose low- and nonfat dairy foods to keep saturated fat intake low. (Most are now available in low-lactose varieties, for those who need them.) Combined with other foods, they can really liven things up. (Think a bit of piquant cheese on vegetables or a dollop of yogurt topping a fruit salad.)

But more than three out of four women don't eat enough dairy foods to ensure proper intake of calcium and all the other nutrients dairy provides. We urge you to shoot for *three servings of low- or nonfat dairy foods daily.* It doesn't just have to be a glass of skim or 1 percent milk or some milk in your cereal. Grate some hard cheese, such as Swiss, cheddar, or Muenster, over the top of a casserole. (If you don't buy reduced-fat hard cheese, you'll want to make especially sure to use cheese as a condiment or to accent a dish rather than as a meal centerpiece because while it's high in calcium and other minerals and vitamins, it's also high in saturated fat.) Or sprinkle plain yogurt with muesli and sunflower or pumpkin seeds or mix it with fresh or frozen fruit.

You can also mix into yogurt dried cherries, golden raisins, dried cranberries, or any other dried fruit that suits your fancy (for wonderful flavor and texture, mix it in the night before). And mozzarella sticks, which have a long refrigerator life, are great for snacks and travel well.

Finally, sandwiches made with low-fat cheese are helped along with some fine mustard and thick slices of ripe tomato.

Target Heart-Healthy Proteins

GOAL: three to four servings daily

SERVING SIZE: 3 ounces cooked fish

½ cup cooked beans

½ cup tofu

1 egg

2 tablespoons peanut butter

3 ounces cooked, skinless poultry

3 ounces cooked lean beef, pork, or lamb

By heart-healthy proteins, we mean proteins that don't come coupled with a lot of saturated fat, which some sources of protein do, including fatty cuts of meat and full-fat dairy products.

High on our list of good-for-your-heart proteins is fish. You can certainly follow a heart-healthy eating plan without eating any fish, but if you're not a vegetarian, we urge you to eat *at least two fish meals a week*. The evidence is overwhelming that including some fish in the diet helps stave off heart disease. Of course, fish that are rich in omega-3 fatty acids, including salmon (wild *or* farmed), mackerel, and herring, are particularly good for your heart (they tend to have darker-colored flesh). But we don't want you to get hung up on the type of fish you eat. It's more important, especially if you're not a fish eater currently, simply to begin to incorporate more fish into your diet. Even tuna sandwiches count—but frozen fish sticks, fried clams, and fried, breaded shrimp do not. With those choices, the actual amount of fish tends to be rather meager, and the type of cooking fat used tends to be high in *trans-* or saturated fatty acids. The cooking method should keep fat and salt on the relatively low side. The best bets are baked or broiled fish. Not only will they be heart-healthy, but they will also be replacing heart-*un*healthy choices you may have otherwise opted for, say, pasta in cream sauce or a hamburger.

Dr. Lichtenstein Talks Safe Fish

You may have read or heard news reports that some types of fish are high in mercury and contaminants called PCBs. But it's not as dangerous as it may sound. In fact, the Food and Drug Administration has issued specific guidelines for only four types of fish: shark, swordfish, king mackerel, and tilefish. Furthermore, the advisory for these rarely eaten fish is only for women of childbearing years as well as young children. Those groups should not eat any fish from those species. They can eat up to 12 ounces a week—four to six servings— of any other fish except canned white albacore tuna. It has more mercury than canned light tuna, so women of childbearing age and children should eat no more than one 6-ounce can of white albacore a week.

For all other people, there are no fish species that are off limits. Vary the type of fish you eat, as your taste dictates.

As you consider fish, keep in mind the risk/benefit ratio. Your risk of developing cardiovascular disease is relatively high in the scheme of things, and the evidence is quite consistent that eating fish on a regular basis reduces that risk. Your risk of mercury toxicity or toxicity of other contaminants, on the other hand, is quite low. When put into perspective, the choice to include fish in the diet is a no-brainer.

For specific questions regarding the safety of eating different fish, go to www.fda.gov, or call the Food and Drug Administration at 1–888–SAFEFOOD.

We want to point out here that even the staunchest non–fish eater can be converted. Alice's teenage daughter turned up her nose at fish until one of her friends brought a tuna sandwich to school with just a little bit of mayo, plenty of curry, and a few raisins. She liked it so much that the "no fish" barrier was broken. Now she will even eat flounder. So experiment for yourself and your family.

Beans are a great protein source, too. They're one of the few protein sources, in fact, that contain a lot of fiber—up to 8 grams per half cup. And

To Eat Eggs or Not?

A lot of people think eggs are *verboten* if you're trying to protect your heart. They're not. Yes, they are high in dietary cholesterol. But as we said in chapter 4, we now know that while the cholesterol in food can raise blood cholesterol, saturated fat and *trans*-fatty acids generally raise blood cholesterol—and heart disease risk—considerably more. The amount of cholesterol in your food doesn't correlate with the amount of cholesterol in your bloodstream.

We don't mean that limiting dietary cholesterol isn't important. Both the National Heart, Lung, and Blood Institute's National Cholesterol Education Program and the American Heart Association advise that you limit dietary cholesterol to an average of 300 milligrams a day for healthy people (200 milligrams if you already have heart disease).

An egg yolk (where all the cholesterol resides in an egg) has about 215 milligrams. Meat, fish, and full-fat dairy foods have some cholesterol, too. Three ounces of cooked chicken, for instance, contains some 65 milligrams, and an ounce of Swiss cheese has 26. So you have to be thoughtful if you want to eat an egg every single day and stay within the 300-milligram limit. But certainly, you could fit in several eggs a week and not exceed the recommendations. For a lower-cholesterol option, you can substitute two egg whites for one whole egg or use the egg substitutes that are available in the supermarket freezer section.

they contain virtually no saturated fat! Always keep a large variety of canned beans in the cupboard or pantry so that you can use them creatively at mealtimes. Throw them into tossed salads, add to vegetable stir-fries and to your favorite soup, or simply have them as a side dish.

Beef, pork, and chicken are fine on our heart-healthy plan, too, especially if you broil or grill them because those methods don't add more calories or saturated fat. Just be sure to keep meat portions on the small side. (If you

Savor a Little Alcohol?

Moderate alcohol consumption—which for women is no more than one drink a day—seems to be protective against heart disease. And it doesn't have to be a 3- to 5-ounce glass of red wine. It can be white wine, or a 12-ounce beer or a drink made with an ounce to an ounce and a half of spirits. Red wine does contain phenols, compounds that come from the skin of grapes that have been touted to benefit the heart. But it's the alcohol itself that studies have most consistently linked to a reduced risk for heart disease.

Having said that, we want to make clear that we don't encourage anyone who does not drink to *take up* drinking for the purpose of reducing cardiovascular disease risk. The combined evidence for an eating plan with plenty of vegetables, fruits, and whole grains along with some fish, other heart-healthy protein foods, and low-fat dairy items is much stronger than the evidence for alcohol, which for some people can be addictive. Moreover, even moderate alcohol intake has been associated with an increased risk for breast cancer—something women at high risk for that disease need to take into consideration when deciding whether to drink. Furthermore, if a woman of childbearing years becomes pregnant and continues to drink, harm to the fetus may occur.

Finally, it needs to be taken into consideration that a glass of wine, a drink made with spirits, or a beer contains anywhere from 100 to 200 calories. That, combined with the potential for alcohol abuse (it's not just a man's problem), should give further pause.

have 6 ounces of chicken, that's two protein servings.) And when it comes to meat, look for lean cuts—generally, ones that have the words "round" or "loin" in their names. Those are the cuts that tend to be lower in saturated fat. To keep down saturated fat in *ground* beef, buy at least 93 percent lean (although no ground beef is truly very lean, even though the numbers might suggest otherwise).

One way to stretch meat or chicken is with a stir-fry. Neither of us normally uses a recipe. Try the following: Sauté a little sliced onion in vegetable oil. When soft (but not brown), add thinly sliced pieces of meat. When the pink is gone, scoop out the meat and add thinly sliced vegetables to the pan—anything from summer squash and peppers to snow peas, green beans, mushrooms, and cauliflower or broccoli florets. Sauté the vegetables until they're wilted. Add the meat back in, stir to heat through again, and serve over brown rice.

This same stir-fry template works for extra-firm tofu, high in protein but virtually devoid of saturated fat. The smallish chunks of tofu you cut from a block should brown on the outside edges before you scoop them up from the pan.

Another delicious way to use tofu is to put it in the food processor with sesame seed paste, lemon juice, and cumin to taste. If you use silken (rather than firm) tofu, it makes a great vegetable dip, salad dressing, or spread.

BRINGING THE "HEART" ACRONYM TO YOUR TABLE

We believe very strongly that each woman needs to tailor a heart-healthy pattern of eating to her own tastes. But sometimes it's hard to get started. You can know everything you're supposed to do but still have a hard time putting it all together. Hence, the sample eating plan below. It will give you a feel for how all the research comes together to form a heart-healthy dietary pattern.

The plan below will also help you turn on the "switch" in your head that will allow you to move forward with better eating. Behavior change can be hard, but with a template that you can tailor to your own preferences, you're one step closer to your heart-healthy eating goal.

Each day's worth of food ranges from about 1,400 to 1,700 calories, including a mandatory fruit snack. If you choose an additional snack or two, it ranges up to 2,000 calories. (Of course, if you want a larger portion at a meal, cut down somewhere else during the day, or perhaps on the snacks.) You can mix and match breakfasts, lunches, and dinners as you see fit. There isn't any magic to the order in which they are presented because it's never about one or another particular food. It's the overall pattern that makes the difference. Also, this is not a weight-loss plan. If you need to lose weight, you will need to pay particular attention to the serving sizes and opt for fewer snacks (and carefully review chapter 7).

BREAKFAST

Option 1: "Pick and Choose"   Amount

GRAIN (TWO OF THE FOLLOWING OR A DOUBLE SERVING)

Whole-grain cold cereal (see package for serving size)	½ to 1 cup
Whole-grain hot cereal (oatmeal, kasha, wheatberries, etc.)	½ cup
Whole-grain bread (toasted or plain)	1 (1-oz.) slice
Whole-grain bagel or English muffin	1 ounce

FRUIT (ONE OF THE FOLLOWING—FRESH, FROZEN, OR CANNED)

Whole, fresh fruit (apple, peach, banana, orange, etc.)	1 medium
Whole, fresh fruit (berries, grapes, etc.)	1 cup
Sliced or chopped fruit (melon, peach, etc.)	1 cup fresh or ½ cup frozen
Dried fruit (apricots, prunes, cranberries, etc.)	¼ cup
100% juice	¾ cup

DAIRY (ONE OF THE FOLLOWING)

Milk (skim or 1%)	1 cup
Yogurt (low- or nonfat)	6 to 8 ounces
Hard cheese (cheddar, Swiss, etc.)	1 ounce

Low-fat hard cheese	1½ ounces
Ricotta cheese (part-skim)	½ cup
Cottage cheese (1% fat or nonfat)	½ cup

Option 2: "Egg Breakfast"

Omelet (in nonstick pan with vegetable oil spray)	3 egg whites or equivalent egg substitute
Vegetables (sautéed in 1 teaspoon vegetable oil)	½ cup
Whole-grain toast (or other grain from above)	1 (1-oz.) slice
One dairy from above	
One fruit from above	

Breakfast: 300 to 400 calories

LUNCH

Option 1: "Classic Sandwich"   Amount

Whole-grain bread	2 (1-oz.) slices
Lean protein (fish, chicken, turkey, beef)	2 ounces
Vegetables (whatever you prefer)	½ cup
Mayonnaise (reduced fat) and/or mustard	1 tablespoon
One dairy from above	

Note: If you prefer to have two portions of lean protein in your sandwich, omit the dairy; if you prefer to have two portions of dairy, omit the lean protein.

Option 2: "Hearty Soup"

Hearty soup (non-cream-based vegetable with beans or meat, such as minestrone)	1½ cups
Whole-wheat bread (pita or equivalent)	1 to 2 (1-oz.) portions
One dairy from above	

Option 3: "Zesty Salad"

Lettuce greens (variety)	2 cups
Fish, chicken, cheese, or tofu (minimally processed)	2 ounces fish or chicken, 1 ounce cheese, ½ cup tofu
Vegetables (variety, chopped)	½ to 1 cup
Dressing (vegetable oil–based)	2 tablespoons
Whole-wheat bread (pita or equivalent)	1 (1-oz.) portion
One dairy from above	

Note: If you prefer to have two portions of lean protein in your salad, omit the dairy; if you prefer to have two portions of dairy, omit the lean protein.

FRUIT
All three lunch options include a fruit serving (see page 81 for serving sizes).

Lunch: 500 to 600 calories

SNACK

To make your diet nutritionally complete, you should include a fruit as a snack at least once during the day (see page 81 for serving sizes).

DINNER

Option 1: "Traditional"   Amount

Lean meat (fish, chicken, beef, pork, lamb), baked, broiled, grilled, or poached	3 ounces
Sauce (barbeque, teriyaki, etc.), optional	2 tablespoons

STARCH (CHOOSE ONE FROM BELOW)
Rice (preferably brown)	½ cup
Pasta (preferably whole wheat)	½ cup

Other whole grain (wheatberries,
  kasha, barley, etc.)   ½ cup
Potato (with 2 tablespoons light sour cream)   1 small

Vegetables (sautéed, grilled, roasted
  with 1 teaspoon vegetable oil)   ½ to 1 cup
Tossed salad (mixture of lettuce and
  other vegetables)   2 cups
Dressing (vegetable oil–based)   2 tablespoons

Option 2: "One Dish"

Vegetable lasagna (with part-skim
  ricotta cheese)   3-by-4-inch rectangle

(Or any other one-dish meal such as: baked ziti mixed with sautéed vegetables and topped with part-skim mozzarella cheese; or taco with chicken, vegetables, and shredded low-fat cheddar cheese. Serving size no greater than 1 cup or 3-by-4-inch rectangle.)

Tossed salad (mixture of lettuce
  and other vegetables)   2 cups
Dressing (vegetable oil–based)   2 tablespoons

Option 3: "Vegan"

Tofu (extra-firm) or veggie burger   ½ cup or 1 patty
Green leafy vegetable (spinach,
  kale, broccoli, etc.)   ½ cup
Rice (brown)   ½ cup
Beans (kidney, black, etc.)   ½ cup
Tossed salad (mixture of lettuce
  and other vegetables)   2 cups
Dressing (vegetable oil–based)   2 tablespoons

Dinner: 500 to 600 calories

A Note About Calories

Calorie ranges for three meals and a mandatory snack, using the tight portion sizes noted above, is 1,400 to 1,700 calories. The reality is there tends to be some drift upward in portion sizes and ingredient variations that can add calories. Thus, the most likely scenario is that this eating pattern will put you closer to 1,700 calories a day rather than 1,400. Everybody's calorie needs are different; therefore, you may find that you need to adjust the serving sizes.

ADDITIONAL SNACK IDEAS

Depending upon your calorie needs, you may be having more than just the single mandatory snack each day. If so, choose from the list below.

Snack Options	Amount
Baby carrots or other raw vegetable with optional dip (see recipe)	10 baby carrots or ½ cup raw vegetables and ⅛ to ¼ cup dip
Yogurt or milk (nonfat, nonsugared)	6 to 8 ounces
Hard cheese	1 ounce
Low-fat hard cheese (cheese sticks)	1½ ounces
Nuts (dry, raw, or roasted, low-sodium)	3 tablespoons
Fruit (without added sugar)	1 small to medium or ½ cup frozen or canned, or 1 cup fresh

Each snack provides roughly 80 to 120 calories.

Coffee or tea are okay at each meal with skim or 1% milk and no more than 1 teaspoon of sugar *or* artificial sweetener.

Where Do Treats Fit In?

You may have noticed that we did not include in the food choices any ice cream, cake, cookies, chips, and so on. We do not mean to say that you

Portion Primer

We cannot stress enough how important it is for you to be aware of portion sizes. Portion sizes in the United States have increased greatly in the last thirty years. Even plates in restaurants are bigger, as are cup holders in cars; eating (and drinking!) more and more over time is a very insidious process.

Most people aren't accustomed to thinking carefully enough about portions, even though they know that portion size counts. It's all too simple to forget that a dash of half-and-half in coffee can easily become 3 tablespoons at 20 calories each; or that a dribble of maple syrup on pancakes becomes 4 tablespoons, or more than 200 calories' worth. Similarly, a pasta meal with breadsticks at an Italian restaurant can easily contain enough grain servings to feed four.

You can balance this—without becoming obsessive. You just need to reeducate yourself about what a proper portion is. Some seem ridiculously small. But that is because they are simply units of measurement, not necessarily amounts that you might normally eat in one sitting.

In this chapter we give the portion sizes for the various food categories. We urge you to measure and weigh your food for a couple of weeks to familiarize yourself with them. Use (and buy if you don't yet have them) a set of measuring cups, measuring spoons, and a food scale. What seems like 3 ounces of chicken breast could easily be 6, and what seems like a 40-calorie teaspoon of cooking oil could easily be a 180-calorie tablespoon and a half. The same goes for a half cup of cooked rice or spaghetti. Volume piles on fast. As for baked goods, look at the label or use a scale. Most muffins, bagels, and even many slices of bread are larger than 1 ounce. Measure what you normally eat. Once you develop an eye for size, volume, and weight, you won't have to keep measuring. You'll know automatically how much breakfast cereal is a serving, how much meat is a 3-ounce portion, and so on. It doesn't mean you can never have two or more portions at once. You can, as long as you don't go over the recommended daily total.

Every six months or so, do a reality check with your measuring utensils. You'd be amazed at how easy it is to drift upward again when you think portion sizes are staying the same.

should never eat them. But, just like when we were kids, they do not have to be on the menu seven days a week. A cookie or two a couple of times a week is fine. A half cup of ice cream occasionally—also no problem. It's when sweets and salty snacks start to become part of the dietary pattern rather than the exception that a heart-healthy diet veers too far off course.

Portion size is a concern here, too. Try to keep portion sizes of treats on the modest side. Use whatever strategy works. Some people keep mini Halloween-size candy bars in the house and are able to limit themselves to one. Others can keep it to one or two cookies at a time. If "in the house" is too close, treat yourself to a frozen yogurt at an ice cream shop once in a while so that you don't always have it tempting you from the kitchen freezer.

SEVEN STRONG HEARTS MENUS

You can actually create any number of menus that suit your fancy from the breakfast, lunch, dinner, and snack options we have suggested. However you use these items, the pattern will be right. What follows are merely suggestions. Use them, tweak them, or ignore them as you see fit—as long as you make sure to choose from the patterns we recommend above, always staying within portion-size guidelines, especially if weight control is a concern.

◉ *WELCOMING SPRING* ◉

Breakfast
Yogurt (plain, nonfat) topped with low-sugar granola spiked with
sunflower and pumpkin seeds and dried chopped apricots
Navel orange

Lunch
Hearty tossed salad with sliced grilled chicken
Oil and vinegar
Whole-wheat pita with tomato and mustard with slice of cheddar cheese
Ripe pear

Afternoon snack
Fresh strawberries

Dinner
Tossed green salad
Citrus-Grilled Salmon (see recipe)
Fusili pasta with a dash of olive oil and garlic and
freshly grated Parmesan cheese
Steamed asparagus

Optional second and third snacks; see snack list for suggestions.

◉ *SUMMER VACATION* ◉

Breakfast
Bran flakes topped with milk
Fresh blueberries

Lunch
Curried Tuna Salad Sandwich with lettuce (see recipe)
Whole-wheat pita
Wedge of watermelon

Afternoon Snack
Fresh raspberries and vanilla yogurt

Dinner
Garden salad
Barbecued chicken breast
Small baked potato topped with light sour cream and sprinkle of chives
Grilled summer squash and zucchini brushed with olive oil

Optional second and third snacks; see snack list for suggestions.

◉ *EMBRACING FALL* ◉

Breakfast
Toasted whole-grain English muffin topped with 1% cottage cheese
Half grapefruit

Lunch
Black Bean Salad with Tomato, Avocado, and Lime Dressing (see recipe)
Crusty French bread
Ripe peach

Afternoon Snack
McIntosh apple

Dinner
Fresh spinach, tomato, and part-skim-milk mozzarella salad
Roasted turkey breast
Roasted root vegetables (carrots, turnips, sweet potato)
drizzled with balsamic vinegar

Optional second and third snacks; see snack list for suggestions.

◎ CELEBRATING WINTER ◎

Breakfast
Steel-cut oatmeal with dried cranberries
Low- or nonfat milk
Half grapefruit

Lunch
Hearty chicken, barley, and vegetable soup
Crusty Tuscan whole-wheat bread with Havarti cheese
Clementine

Afternoon Snack
Gala apple

Dinner
Tossed salad with balsamic vinaigrette dressing
Grilled lean sirloin steak
Wheatberry Salad (see recipe)
Roasted brussels sprouts with Vidalia onions

Optional second and third snacks; see snack list for suggestions.

◎ WEEKEND FARE ◎

Breakfast
Vegetable-and-cheese omelet
Whole-wheat toast
Fresh-squeezed orange juice

Lunch
Caesar salad with grated Parmesan cheese
Rye crispbread
Plum

Afternoon Snack
Pineapple

Dinner
Tossed salad
Baked Flounder with Lemon Sauce (see recipe)
Rice pilaf
Steamed carrots and green beans

Optional second and third snacks; see snack list for suggestions.

◎ A VEGETARIAN AFFAIR ◎

Breakfast
Muesli with dried fruit and nuts
Low- or nonfat milk or soymilk

Lunch
Lentil soup
Whole-wheat bread with Swiss cheese, shredded lettuce, and zesty mustard
Tomato and cucumber salad with olive oil
Red grapes

Afternoon snack
Honeydew melon and cantaloupe

Dinner
Tossed summer salad with vinaigrette dressing
Vegetable tofu stir-fry with seasonal vegetables
Brown rice
Black beans

Optional second and third snacks; see snack list for suggestions.

❂ *WEEKDAY FARE* ❂

Breakfast
Puffed-wheat cereal with skim milk
Blueberries and strawberries

Lunch
Mixed green salad with sliced chicken breast, vegetables, feta cheese,
olives, cherry tomatoes and vinaigrette dressing
Whole-wheat pita
Nectarine

Afternoon Snack
Fruit smoothie with nonfat yogurt

Dinner
Shrimp and vegetable stir-fry (snow peas, onions,
garlic, mushrooms, and peppers)
Whole-wheat couscous

Optional second and third snacks; see snack list for suggestions.

STRONG WOMEN, STRONG HEARTS RECIPES

All the recipes listed below, which go with many of the menus you might
want to create, are ones we both use—and love. (If we don't like it, we don't
eat it—and we suggest you follow that guideline, too.)

CITRUS-GRILLED SALMON

(Four servings)

This is a simple yet delicious way to prepare heart-healthy salmon.

Nonstick cooking spray, or 1 tablespoon olive oil
2 lemons
2 limes
4 cloves garlic
Freshly ground pepper (to taste)
1 pound salmon fillets

Heat the grill to medium-high. Spray a large piece of aluminum foil with nonstick cooking spray and turn it up along the edges. Cut the lemons and limes in half and squeeze all of the juice into a large measuring cup, being careful to filter any seeds. Peel and chop the garlic. Then whisk the juice, garlic, and pepper together. Pour about one-quarter of the mixture into the aluminum foil; place the fish on top; pour the rest of the liquid over the fish. Loosely wrap it up, folding over the foil to keep the moisture in while grilling but with enough openings for the juice to (mostly) evaporate. Grill for about 5 minutes on one side and then open the foil to flip the fish once midway through, for a total of 10 to 15 minutes until cooked through (time will vary, depending on grill temperature and thickness of the fish). Cut into four pieces.

BAKED FLOUNDER WITH LEMON SAUCE

(Four servings)

Here is a quick way to dress up a mild fish.

2 tablespoons low-fat plain yogurt
2 tablespoons reduced-fat mayonnaise
1 tablespoon lemon juice
Fresh dill, chopped
1 pound flounder fillet

Preheat oven to 400°F. Mix yogurt, mayonnaise, lemon juice, and dill together. Spread sauce over flounder fillet. Bake for about 10 minutes or until fish flakes. Do not overcook.

CURRIED TUNA

(Two servings)

This is Alice's daughter's favorite recipe for tuna. It is quick and delicious.

One 6-ounce can tuna (packed in water), drained
1 tablespoon reduced-fat mayonnaise
1 teaspoon curry, or to taste
3 tablespoons raisins
3 tablespoons slivered almonds

Break up tuna pieces with a fork, mix in mayonnaise, add remaining ingredients, toss.

Variation: Add one medium-size diced apple or ½ cup chopped celery.

BLACK BEAN SALAD WITH TOMATO, AVOCADO, AND LIME DRESSING

◆

(Three to four servings)

This recipe is from Miriam's book Strong Women Eat Well *and was created by her collaborator, Judy Knipe. It is a good, quick recipe that is perfect for ripe avocados. Eat the salad the same day you make it—before the avocado changes color.*

One 15-ounce can black beans
½ cup diced red onion
½ cup diced green or red bell pepper
½ jalapeño pepper, cored, seeded, and minced (optional)
½ cup quartered grape or cherry tomatoes
½ ripe avocado, diced
2 tablespoons chopped fresh coriander

Dressing

2 tablespoons fresh lime juice
1 teaspoon sherry vinegar
1 tablespoon extra-virgin olive oil
½ teaspoon ground cumin
Salt to taste
Freshly ground black pepper

Drain the beans, rinse them very briefly under cold running water, and drain again. Transfer them to a bowl, add onion, bell pepper, jalapeño pepper (if using), tomato, avocado, and coriander, and toss lightly.

Combine all the dressing ingredients in a small bowl and whisk until well mixed. Add the dressing to the bean mixture and stir gently. Cover the salad with waxed paper or plastic wrap and allow the flavors to blend for 1 or 2 hours at room temperature or in the refrigerator. Bring the salad back to room temperature before serving.

WHEATBERRIES WITH DRIED CRANBERRIES AND HONEY-ORANGE DRESSING

(Makes 3½ to 4 cups; serving size ½ cup)

This recipe is also adapted from Miriam's book Strong Women Eat Well. *Her colleague Judy Knipe introduced her to wheatberries with this dish. It is a staple in Miriam's house now. The entire family loves it. The wheatberries cook up to a beautiful pale color and a tender but crunchy texture. The dish is delicious served by itself but can also be served for breakfast topped with yogurt or as an accompaniment to meats, fish, and poultry.*

  1 cup summer (soft) wheatberries
  ½ cup orange juice
  4 teaspoons honey
  6 tablespoons pine nuts
  ¼ cup dried cranberries, coarsely chopped
  Salt to taste

Pour wheatberries into a heavy, medium-size saucepan, add water to cover by an inch or two, and bring to a boil. Cover the pan, turn to low, and simmer the berries, covered, for about 2 hours or until the grain is cooked but still crunchy. (The berries cook faster if you soak them overnight.) Drain the wheatberries and transfer to a bowl. You will have a generous 2½ cups.

Mix together the orange juice and honey. Add the sweetened juice to the wheatberries and toss together with the pine nuts and chopped cranberries. Mix well and taste for salt, which, added in very small amounts, brings out the flavor of the fruit.

Serve warm, at room temperature, or cold.

CLASSIC VINAIGRETTE DRESSING

◊

Miriam *learned how to prepare this dressing in a cooking class while studying abroad during college.*

⅔ cup of good-quality olive oil
⅓ cup balsamic vinegar
1 teaspoon dried basil, or 1 tablespoon fresh
1 tablespoon French mustard
½ teaspoon sugar
½ teaspoon salt
Pepper to taste

Pour into a salad dressing decanter, insert stopper, and shake vigorously.

SUMMER CUCUMBER DIP

◊

(Makes 3 cups; serving size 2 tablespoons)

This *dip is the perfect complement for baby carrots, peppers, or other vegetables.*

½ cucumber
2 cups plain nonfat yogurt
½ teaspoon salt
2 cloves garlic, crushed
1 tablespoon olive oil

Peel, seed, and shred the cucumber. In a colander, press the liquid out of the cucumber. Mix the yogurt, salt, garlic, and olive oil in a bowl, stir in the cucumber, and serve.

CHAPTER 6

The Right Exercises for Optimal Heart Health

◆

As I got older, I wanted to make sure I wasn't going to get heart disease. I also knew that it was going to get harder and harder to maintain my weight. But my exercise had always been episodic. I'm talking four to six times a year.

For me, the logical way to get into it was to join a gym, but I couldn't bring myself to go because I was so incredibly intimidated by all the machines and weights. I was resisting because I was embarrassed and rationalizing that I didn't have time. Finally, I went to the local Y. I decided to go on Saturday mornings. I knew I should be doing this several times a week, but you've got to start somewhere.

When I first got there, I was relieved, first of all, because people were in sweats. It wasn't like they were all wearing Lycra. Also, they were all shapes, sizes, and ages. I had thought no gym would ever have a person like me—a woman in her fifties who's not a trained athlete and doesn't have a perfect figure. Plus, a trainer spent an entire hour with me, showing me how to use the machines. This was routine. It had never occurred to me that they would do this.

Three years ago, I couldn't have imagined walking into a gym and using any of the machines. I never thought about my "abs." I am now 100 percent committed.

—HELEN

A long with good, wholesome nutrition, there is no more important thing you can do for your heart than move your body—get your heart rate up, use your muscles, and expend more energy. But a regular exercise routine does a lot more than protect your heart. It also improves outlook; increases bone density; ups your energy level; retards the muscle atrophy and creeping frailty that occur as we age; and is crucial, as you will learn in the next chapter, for weight control. Says Helen, "I have not gained weight since menopause, as some of my friends have."

There are two types of physical activity that we encourage you to incorporate into your lifestyle: aerobic activity and strength training. On top of those two kinds of planned exercise, we hope you will engage in something we call *decreasing sedentary living*—using your body to move through the day in a way you might not have been doing until now, especially if you work a desk job or don't go out much.

Even with the different activities combined, we're only talking about three to six hours a week. We understand that your schedule might already be packed and that you feel you can't possibly see your way to incorporating something new into your calendar. But what we both have heard over and over again is that while a woman might feel tired for the first couple of weeks after she starts an exercise program, a physical activity regime so enhances a person's energy level and feelings of well-being that she soon doesn't know how she was able to go for so many years *without* regular exercise. As Helen describes it, "I can walk up five flights of stairs now and not even think about it. I can jog three miles on a treadmill instead of walking a mile or two. It's easier to carry heavy things. I don't get back pain anymore when I sit at the computer."

Following is a step-by-step plan for making the different prongs of our exercise program a part of your life. At all points we emphasize *gradual* adaptation to increased physical activity. Try to tackle too much too fast, and you'll end up exhausted, achy, and uncomfortable. Add to your exercise routine in a slow, deliberate manner, and within just a few weeks you will truly start to feel like a new person. Your heart health will benefit almost immediately, too. Within weeks of beginning an exercise program, blood pressure starts to drop and the heart begins to beat more efficiently. You'll *feel* great, too.

FIRST STEP: DECREASE SEDENTARY LIVING

In the spirit of taking this one sure step at a time, we feel it is very important that before you begin a formal exercise program, you spend two weeks finding ways in your routine to decrease a sedentary lifestyle. You may want to start by engaging in brisk walking and strength training right away, but we guarantee that if you spend just two weeks taking stock of your current level of physical activity and see where you can unobtrusively "insert" more here and there—that is, if you begin by raising your level of activity consciousness—you'll be much more prepared to begin the formal program, and you'll be more likely to succeed.

We're talking about things you've heard a lot about but that few people actually do: taking the stairs instead of the elevator; not driving around the supermarket parking lot to find the space closest to the door but parking instead wherever you first see a space; walking rather than driving to destinations you can reach on foot within ten minutes (which will ensure walking a mile there and back); getting up to turn the television on and off manually rather than using the remote; and so on.

It may not seem like it adds up to much, but it does. You can easily burn an extra 100 calories a day with those small bursts of physical activity—enough to lose 10 excess pounds in a year without eating less. And, of course, every time you move around rather than sit, you challenge your heart to beat a little faster, training it to be stronger and fitter. That is, the more you push your heart and the rest of your cardiovascular system to do, the more they *can* do.

We both engage in exactly the things we're encouraging. It isn't always easy, and we aren't perfect all the time, but overall we are pretty consistent. Alice works on the fifth floor of a research center at Tufts and often walks up to her office rather than taking the elevator. And she rarely uses the elevator to go from floor to floor once she's in the building. Miriam, too, doesn't use the elevator in her eight-story research building a block and a half away. And neither of us wastes time driving around the mall looking for a spot close to the entrance. We also walk or ride our bicycles when we can (Miriam lives 1.5 miles from her town center, Alice, several blocks from her post office) and do not shy away from some of the heavier outdoor work around the house, including raking leaves, shoveling snow, and stacking wood.

Obviously, if you have been sedentary for most or all of your adult life, you should not start trying to decrease your sedentariness by shoveling snow for a half hour or walking up ten flights of stairs to your office. Not only could it dissolve your resolve to push on even before you truly get started, it could also be risky. But just about all women can think of safe ways to incorporate a little more physical activity into their lives here and there, even if it's as simple as taking something upstairs every time you think of it rather than building a pile at the bottom of the stairs to take up in one trip at the end of the day.

You'll be surprised at the end of two weeks how many little "pieces" of physical activity you can tuck into your day without losing a lot of time—or energy. You'll be surprised, too, at the sense of self-confidence you begin to enjoy by using your body more. Furthermore, you'll be more ready to tackle the structured part of our exercise plan, both physically and emotionally.

BEFORE YOU START THE FORMAL PROGRAM

After two weeks of making a concentrated effort to get more physical activity here and there, you might be eager to get the actual exercise sessions under way. Before you do, we strongly advise you to take the PAR-Q (Physical Activity Readiness Questionnaire) that follows.

Most everyone can participate in our exercise program without any problems, but by taking the PAR-Q, you're adding an extra level of caution—never a bad thing. (If you're over 70, the PAR-Q alone will not cut it. We strongly recommend that you see your doctor to get a professional go-ahead before taking up an exercise plan.)

Exercise Clothes, Gear, and Personal Effects
You are going to need to buy some essentials to get you going—both correctly and safely. It'll be a pretty modest investment overall—even more so when you consider the return in health benefits.

Athletic Shoes

Last year Miriam trained for the Boston Marathon as part of a large effort at Tufts called the President's Marathon Challenge. Even she, an accomplished athlete, had a hard time finding the right athletic shoes for her training runs—her feet are very narrow. But she kept at it until she tried on a pair that fit comfortably, had the right stability for her gait, and were light enough for long-distance running.

Admittedly, training for a marathon is different from incorporating a regular program of physical activity into your routine, but either way, the comfort and health of your feet are critical for your success. So choose carefully. Make sure the shoe fits—and also fits the type of exercise in which you plan to participate. (For instance, running shoes tend to be lighter than walking shoes.) And once your athletic shoes are six to nine months old, consider buying a new pair. To check whether your shoes are worn out, place them on a table or counter at eye level and look to see whether the soles are worn on either the outside or the inside edges. That should be the trigger that sends you back to a store where the salespeople have expertise in fitting shoes. Exercising with shoes that are worn out puts too much stress on the joints. That's true for *all* your shoes, not just the ones you work out in.

Dumbbells

Unless you join a fitness center you will need to buy some dumbbells. The strength-training component of the program requires starting with a 3-pound and a 5-pound pair of dumbbells, or hand weights. As you get stronger, you will need pairs of 6-, 8-, 10-, and, in some cases, 12-pound dumbbells, available at sporting good stores and many department stores. (But you can wait until you get to that level to buy those.) Expect to pay about 60 cents a pound.

Some dumbbells are adjustable by weight so you don't have to buy more than one pair. If you go that route, make sure they are comfortable to hold— and easy to adjust.

Staircase, Step, or Utility Stool

One of the exercises requires a step. You need to buy a step or stool *only* if you don't have a staircase at home. You can buy a step for about $50 at a sporting goods store—or a sturdy utility stool 8 to 12 inches high for $10 to

Physical Activity Readiness
Questionnare—PAR-Q
(revised 1994)

PAR-Q & YOU
(A Questionnaire for People Aged 15 to 69)

Regular physical activity is fun and healthy, and increasingly more people are starting to become more active every day. Being more active is very safe for most people. However, some people should check with their doctor before they start becoming much more physically active.

If you are planning to become much more physically active than you are now, start by answering the seven questions in the box below. If you are between the ages of 15 and 69, the PAR-Q will tell you if you should check with your doctor before you start. If you are over 69 years of age, and you are not used to being very active, check with your doctor.

Common sense is your best guide when you answer these questions. Please read the questions carefully and answer each one honestly: check YES or NO.

YES NO

☐   ☐   1. Has your doctor ever said that you have a heart condition *and* that you should only do physical activity recommended by a doctor?

☐   ☐   2. Do you feel pain in your chest when you do physical activity?

☐   ☐   3. In the past month, have you had chest pain when you were not doing physical activity?

☐   ☐   4. Do you lose your balance because of dizziness or do you ever lose consciousness?

☐   ☐   5. Do you have a bone or joint problem that could be made worse by a change in your physical activity?

☐   ☐   6. Is your doctor currently prescribing drugs (for example, water pills) for your blood pressure or heart condition?

☐   ☐   7. Do you know of *any other reason* why you should not do physical activity?

**IF
YOU
ANSWERED**

YES to one or more questions

Talk with your doctor by phone or in person BEFORE you start becoming much more physically active or BEFORE you have a fitness appraisal. Tell your doctor about the PAR-Q and which questions you answered YES.

- You may be able to do any activity you want—as long as you start slowly and build up gradually. Or, you may need to restrict your activities to those which are safe for you. Talk with your doctor about the kinds of activities you wish to participate in and follow his/her advice.
- Find out which community programs are safe and helpful for you.

NO to all questions

If you answered NO honestly to <u>all</u> PAR-Q questions, you can be reasonably sure that you can:

- start becoming much more physically active—begin slowly and build up gradually. This is the safest and easiest way to go.
- take part in a fitness appraisal—this is an excellent way to determine your basic fitness so that you can plan the best way for you to live actively.

DELAY BECOMING MUCH MORE ACTIVE:

- if you are not feeling well because of a temporary illness such as a cold or fever—wait until you feel better; or
- if you are or may be pregnant—talk to your doctor before you start becoming more active.

Please note: If your health changes so that you then answer YES to any of the above questions, tell your fitness or health professional. Ask whether you should change your physical activity plan.

Informed Use of the PAR-Q: The Canadian Society for Exercise Physiology, Health Canada, agents assume no liability for persons who undertake physical activity, and if in doubt after completing this questionnaire, consult your doctor prior to physical activity.

$20. You should be able to find the stool at a hardware store or a good department store. Make sure the stool has four solid legs and a skid-proof top. Make sure, too, that it can hold your body weight easily without tipping over.

Exercise Mat

It may seem superfluous, but a firm exercise mat makes floor exercises more comfortable. Exercise mats are relatively inexpensive (about $18) and easy to store, and they make a real difference. Alternatively, you can use a large bath towel. Either one provides added cushioning.

Tops and Bottoms

Make sure to wear loose, nonrestrictive clothing for comfort and to dress appropriately for the weather. (Wear layers in winter so you can tie an outer layer around your waist if you warm up too much as you're going along.)

The newest quick-dry fabrics available for athletic clothing dry quickly when they get wet. It's a big step in improving comfort while you work out. The wetness doesn't turn cold and stick to your body.

You don't need to buy those clothes right now. You most likely have what you need in your closet. As you get more into the program, you can supplement your workout clothes with what's appropriate. (Or you can drop a nice hint to a friend or family member when your birthday is approaching.)

Sun Protection

Get a hat with a visor to protect your eyes, and sunglasses, too. Also, always use sunscreen. Keep a small container of sunscreen with your water bottle. That way, you won't forget to use it.

Water

Last year, the National Academy of Sciences issued a statement saying that it isn't necessary to follow the popular advice to drink at least eight glasses of water a day but, rather, to drink only when you feel thirsty. Nonetheless, we believe water should be an integral part of your workout gear. Drink some just before and just after your aerobic workouts as well as during strength training. Plenty of fluid will allow your body to perform at its best.

Contrary to what you might see in ads, you do not need a sports drink to rehydrate. You don't need the extra calories, either. Sports drinks are for exercise that is of long duration—more than 1½ hours at a time, or if you are working out for a long time in the heat. Stick to good old H_2O instead.

THE STRONG WOMEN, STRONG HEARTS EXERCISE PROGRAM

We put forth here two different possibilities for exercise programs:

- *Minimal* Heart-Healthy Exercise Program
- *Optimal* Heart-Healthy Exercise Program

To produce meaningful results in your cardiovascular system and reduce your risk of heart disease significantly, your level of exercise should fall somewhere on the spectrum between the two program levels. Minimal is fine, especially as a first step. You get the most bang for your effort by going from being completely sedentary to moderately active. But the more you do, the better shape your heart will be in.

Minimal Exercise Program at a Glance

Aerobics:	30 minutes at a time, three days a week, or 15 minutes at a time, six days a week
Flexibility (Stretching):	5 minutes following every exercise session

Optimal Exercise Program at a Glance

Aerobics:	30 or more minutes at a time, five to six days a week
Strength training:	30 minutes at a time, two to three days a week
Flexibility (Stretching):	5 minutes following every exercise session

For some of you, the programs may look daunting. You may never have exercised regularly before, or it may be a long time since you did. For that reason, we cannot emphasize enough that the key to long-term success is to take it slowly but deliberately. At all points, our program encourages you to increase the duration and intensity of your exercise *a little bit at a time.* That will keep you from burning out—and injuring yourself. And for the aerobic exercises, in particular, choose exercises that you enjoy. That's also crucial for sticking with the program.

If you *are* starting from scratch, don't go for thirty minutes of aerobics all at once. Start with short bouts (ten to fifteen minutes in duration) and only half the strength-training routine and work up from there. The most important thing is *consistency.* Don't tell yourself not to bother because you can't do much to start. Keep building on it little by little, individualizing the program so that you stay committed, and continue to build on what you've accomplished.

No matter what your initial level of activity and how slowly you proceed, in just a couple of weeks your endurance and strength will increase. Within six weeks, added vigor and vitality will kick in.

Most women choose brisk walking because you don't have to go to a gym to do it and because everybody knows how to walk. It's not something you have to learn or get better at. But if you really love swimming or biking or some other form of aerobics, go for it. Or cross-train by doing some brisk walking combined with another aerobic activity.

Cross-training might be best for someone who likes to swim or exercise on a bicycle. Walking and running, unlike swimming and biking, are weight-bearing exercises, meaning you carry the weight of your body as you perform the activity. They have an added advantage in that, unlike activities in which you sit or are carried by water, they help maintain the strength of your bones.

Warming Up and Cooling Down

One last bit of preparation before you begin the actual program. Most exercise injuries result from the body (muscles and connective tissue, specifically) not being warmed up or cooled down adequately. To warm up and avoid hurting yourself, do three to five minutes of low-intensity walking, dancing, calisthenics, or riding of a stationary bike before you actually begin the exercise. Many people like to do a milder version of the activity they plan to engage in: walking before running, for instance, or cycling slowly before going at it with greater intensity. A low-intensity warm-up increases muscle and tendon elasticity—the "rubber bands" of your body will have more give—and that in turn decreases the chances of one of them "snapping." Your heart and the rest of your vascular system will also be ready for the workout; they won't have to go into high gear all at once.

A proper cooldown is just as critical for safe exercising. It allows your body to return *slowly* to its resting state. Your heart rate will decrease gradually, as

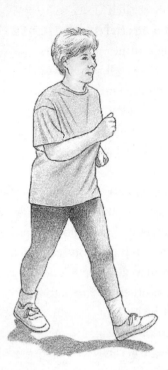

will your blood pressure, easing stress on your system. And, when you cool down properly, the blood in your legs will slowly be shifted back to the rest of your body. Five minutes of light activity—the other "bookend" around your exercise session—will suffice as a cooldown.

If your exercise session is strength training rather than aerobics, a good cooldown is stretching, which takes care of cooling down and flexibility at the same time.

The Aerobic Component

To get heart-healthy results from aerobic exercise, which directly targets the heart, lungs, and the rest of the cardiovascular system, the key is working out at the appropriate *intensity* for a long enough *duration* to make a difference. If you go at it too easily, you won't experience enough improvement. (Going at it too hard can cause injuries and do your heart more harm than good, although

At Home or at the Fitness Center?

Some people prefer exercising at home because of the convenience, the privacy, and the lack of a membership fee. Others prefer having an exercise buddy to keep them motivated. Still others prefer a gym or community center because they can get instruction and guidance from professionals and also use weights *or* resistance machines to vary their strength-training sessions. Some people are lucky enough to have fitness centers at their places of work. It doesn't matter where you exercise. Just make sure it's a place you feel comfortable. There's no point in joining a gym that's either out of the way or filled with members who make you feel intimidated (although, like Helen, you might be surprised to find that a lot of people joining gyms these days look just like you). You'll just end up talking yourself out of going more times than not.

If it's instruction that you need, another option is to spring for a personal trainer at home. They can be expensive—up to $100 an hour—but a few sessions may be all you need to get you started, and to ensure you're using the proper form and technique. A personal trainer can also help you become and stay motivated.

that very rarely occurs. The overwhelming majority of people, when they err, err on the side of not pushing themselves hard enough.)

Determining the Right Intensity

When it is working at its hardest, your heart can beat a certain maximum number of beats per minute. But that's too much for regular exercise, even exercise that lasts only a short while. The right intensity, or range, for exercise is generally 60 to 80 percent of your maximum heart rate. It's safe yet rigorous enough to bring your cardiovascular system to the next level. How do you figure out your maximum heart rate so you can determine 60 to 80 percent of it? It's simple.

Maximum Heart Rate = 220 Minus Your Age

The equation is not perfect. It doesn't take into account variations from person to person. But it's a reasonable ballpark measure that you can use in conjunction with how you feel as you're going along. In other words, if you're exercising at 80 percent of your maximum heart rate but feel like you can't get in enough air or keep up the pace, you'll want to take it down a little.

The following chart gives heart rates—beats per minute—for 60, 70, 80, and 90 percent intensity for a number of ages based on five-year intervals. If your age is not one of the five-year marks, subtract it from 220 and multiply it by 0.60, 0.70, 0.80, and 0.90. That will give you the range of target heart rates for your age.

Target Heart Rate = 60 to 80 percent of Maximun Heart Rate

	HEART RATE IN BEATS PER MINUTE AT DIFFERENT PERCENTS OF MAXIMUM			
AGE	60%	70%	80%	90%
20	120	140	160	180
25	117	137	156	176
30	114	133	152	171
35	111	130	148	167
40	108	126	144	162
45	105	123	140	158
50	102	119	136	153
55	99	116	132	149
60	96	112	128	144
65	93	109	124	140
70	90	105	120	135
75	87	102	116	131
80	84	98	112	126

Of course, once you learn the range for your target heart rate, you need to be able to determine whether you are in that range while you're actually exercising. There are two ways to do that. One is to take your pulse. The other is to use an intensity scale. Many exercisers use a combination of both.

Taking Your Pulse

To take your pulse, hold out your right hand. Press together the index finger and middle finger of your left hand and touch them to the inside of the base of your wrist, just past where your hand ends. Slide your fingers across your right wrist, pressing firmly when you're at the hollow next to the tendons. If you can't feel your pulse, vary how firmly you're pressing or bend your wrist back slightly. Then, watching a clock with a second hand, count the number of beats for thirty seconds, then multiply by two.

You should check your heart rate when you've been doing aerobic activity for five minutes as well as at the end of your workout session, just before you cool down. That way, you can tell whether you're exercising at a high enough intensity (at least 60 percent of your maximum heart rate) but not too high (more than 80 percent).

Note: You don't have to use your fingers to take your pulse. You can buy a heart rate monitor—a strap worn around your mid-chest that sends a signal to a watch on your wrist that gives a heart rate readout. But while heart rate monitors can be useful, they're expensive—$50 to $200, depending on the model.

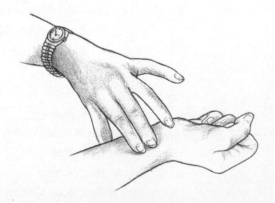

Using the Intensity Scale

Knowing whether you're in the target heart rate range is the most precise way of determining whether you're doing your aerobic exercise at the appropriate intensity. But once you've been exercising for a while and know what it feels like to be in the effective range (this middle ground entails a certain amount of sweating and labored breathing), you can rely more often on the intensity scale. It's a five-point scale, with level 3 corresponding to 60 to 80 percent of your heart rate maximum and occasionally going up to 4.

At level 3, you should more or less be able to keep up a conversation. At level 4, you can complete a couple of sentences here and there. If you can't utter more than a word or two at a time, you're probably exercising at above 90 percent of your maximum heart rate—an unsafe level.

Note: When it's hot or humid outside, the body has a harder time getting rid of its heat. Therefore, working out at any given intensity can result in heart rates that are 10 to 20 beats higher per minute than usual. Be sure to tone down your activity level a bit to account for this factor.

Don't Overdo

We want your exercise to feel like exercise. But if you have not been doing any aerobic activities, you really want to *start slowly*—maybe just five to ten minutes of an activity at a low intensity. Don't worry about intensity up front. After two or three weeks you can begin to increase it, as well as the time spent exercising. If that feels too drawn out, keep in mind that some people haven't exercised in decades. A few weeks of taking it slow isn't going to make a difference. The point at the beginning is that you've gotten started.

Here's a suggested pattern for increasing your aerobic exercise intensity and duration. Remember, the *minimum* you eventually want to work up to is at least thirty minutes three times a week (or fifteen-minute bouts six times a week). The *optimal* is thirty to sixty minutes five to six times a week.

Week 1	60–70% Maximum Heart Rate	5–10 minutes
Week 2	60–70% Maximum Heart Rate	10 minutes
Week 3	60–70% Maximum Heart Rate	15 minutes
Week 4	60–80% Maximum Heart Rate	15 minutes
Week 5	60–80% Maximum Heart Rate	20 minutes
Week 6 and beyond	60–80% Maximum Heart Rate	30 or more minutes

EXERCISE INTENSITY SCALE FOR AEROBIC TRAINING	
EXERCISE INTENSITY LEVEL	DESCRIPTION OF EFFORT
1. Sedentary	No perceived effort: standing, sitting, or lying down.
2. Active This level contributes to overall health and burns more calories than being sedentary.	Easy, sustainable movement that causes a small increase in heart and breathing rate and doesn't raise a sweat (unless the weather is hot): strolling, gardening, slow dancing, golfing.
3. Moderate training You should exercise at this level to condition your heart and the rest of your cardiovascular system.	Somewhat hard movement that elevates the heart rate to 60 to 70 percent of maximum most of the time, ranging up to 80 percent. Breathing is more rapid, though it's possible to converse with only slightly altered speech; perspiration appears after about 5 to 15 minutes, depending on air temperature.
4. Vigorous training This is a more advanced level of aerobic conditioning that becomes an appropriate goal after exercising for several months.	Hard effort that elevates the heart rate to 70 to 80 percent most of the time, ranging up to 90 percent of maximum. Breathing is more rapid but not labored—it's possible to converse, though faster breathing will cause evident interruptions; perspiration starts within 5 to 10 minutes, depending on air temperature; fatigue increases as the workout continues, and you will feel a need to stop by the end.
5. Overexertion Not recommended!	Excessive effort: heart pounds to the point of discomfort or nausea; breathing is too rapid to permit speech.

A Note About Warm-up and Cooldown

You will not be at your target heart rate the entire time you are doing aerobic exercise. It takes about five minutes to work up to it (the warm-up) and five minutes to slow down before you finish in order to ease your muscles out of their more strenuous work (the cooldown). In other words, you do not have to tack on extra time to your aerobics routine for warm-ups and cooldowns. If you exercise for, say, thirty minutes, ten of those minutes will be warm-up and cooldown and twenty will be you working at your target heart rate. That's fine.

That said, it does get a little trickier if you are doing shorter bouts. You will need to add on a little more time to account for the warm-up and cooldown. That's because you need to be at your target heart rate for at least ten minutes at a stretch to truly strengthen your cardiovascular system.

Remember to Enjoy It!

As we said earlier in this chapter, the best aerobic activities are the ones you enjoy, because they're the ones you'll stick with. Most people choose brisk walking, which is great because it can be done just about anywhere with not much more equipment than a good pair of exercise shoes (that are not worn out). Just keep in mind that the walking shouldn't feel like a stroll, even if you go with a friend. Whether on a sidewalk, in a mall, on hilly terrain, or on a treadmill, it should feel purposeful, as if you are pushing yourself to catch a bus or make a meeting on time. That is, by the time you're finished, you should have got warm enough to have broken into at least a light sweat. (It *is* ladylike to sweat. Health, strength, vigor, and vitality are all part of being feminine.)

Along with walking, many people enjoy doing their weight-bearing aerobic activity on *cross-country ski machines* and *elliptical trainers*. A lot of women, in particular, also like using *stair climbers* and *stair-stepping* machines. In addition to providing a great workout, they target the legs, buttocks, and trunk, which many women want to firm up. Exercise classes ranging from *low-impact aerobics* to *boxing* to *dancing* keep women motivated, too. If you want to dance for exercise—but in privacy—rent or buy a dance exercise video. There are also yoga and tai chi, which we will talk about in greater detail in chapter 8.

Non–weight bearing exercises, as we said earlier, include swimming and biking. (When's the last time you were on a bike? Try it! Just don't forget to

What About a Pedometer?

If you are incorporating more walking into your everyday life as part of your work or errands, etc., pedometers are a great tool for determining whether you are actually getting enough exercise. We highly recommend that you wear one to keep track. Health experts say that optimally, you should be accumulating 10,000 steps each day, and we agree. You might not always reach 10,000; it translates to about 4.5 miles over the course of the day. But whether or not you get to that level on a regular basis, a pedometer is a great motivator. Once you have a number, you have a goal—to increase it. Make sure that you follow the manufacturer's directions when wearing the device. Also, keep in mind that you don't need a fancy one. We like the ones that just count steps and nothing more. They cost $15 to $30. See the Resources section for information on purchasing a pedometer.

wear your helmet.) You can also choose rowing—a great whole-body exercise. Non–weight bearing activities are particularly useful at the start for women with osteoarthritis of the knee or hip because they take pressure off the diseased joints in those body parts. But as you progress, do try to incorporate at least some weight-bearing activities in your exercise routine.

THE STRENGTH TRAINING COMPONENT

While aerobic exercise directly targets the heart, lungs, and the rest of the cardiovascular system, strength training is crucial to heart health because it enhances the effect through whole-body muscle conditioning. There's also evidence that it lowers blood pressure. And it reduces fat around the abdomen, which lowers heart disease risk, too.

As with aerobic activities, the key to strength training is to do it regularly—and at the right intensity. You want to challenge your muscles to the point that they adapt to handling a greater amount of weight and become stronger. If you lift weights that are too light, your muscles will not be stimulated enough to "respond." If you lift weights that are too heavy, you can end up injuring not only your muscles but also the joints and other tissues that surround them.

A key point here—and this differs from aerobic activities—is that you must let your muscles *rest* by not strength-training them two days in a row. For every strength-training day on, a set of muscles has to have *the next day off.* That's why you'll never see a recommendation to strength-train, from us or any other credentialed health expert, four to seven days a week. The American Heart Association recommends strength training two days a week. We think that's perfectly acceptable, but we prefer the American College of Sports Medicine's recommendation: *two to three* days per week. Consistency trumps frequency, however. Strength training two days a week every single week is much better than three days a week for a couple of weeks, then once a week for a few more weeks, etc.

What exactly is involved in a strength-training session? In the particular program we outline here, which targets the entire body—trunk, arms, and legs—there are six exercises. Every single time you do one of the exercises— whether it's lifting dumbbells over your shoulders or raising your chest off the floor while lying facedown—it's called a repetition, or rep. Twelve reps make a set, and you want to do *two sets of each exercise* during each exercise session, with a minute or so of rest between sets.

Determining the Right Strength-Training Intensity

If you can do more than 12 reps easily, you're not challenging your muscles enough. And if you can do only 5 or 6 reps before having to stop, you're pushing your muscles to deal with too much at once. If you're conducting the moves at the right intensity, the weight you're lifting or pushing against should feel moderately heavy as you start (but well within your ability), then feel like it's getting heavier and heavier by the sixth or seventh rep. By the twelfth rep, which you should still be able to do in good form, you should feel like if you don't stop and take a break, you couldn't do another one.

As with aerobic exercise, we have developed a scale for evaluating the intensity of your effort. You should use it to judge your intensity at the end of two sets of 12 reps.

EXERCISE INTENSITY SCALE FOR STRENGTH TRAINING	
EXERCISE INTENSITY LEVEL	DESCRIPTION OF EFFORT
1—Very easy	Too easy to be noticed, like lifting a pencil.
2—Easy	Can be felt but isn't fatiguing, like carrying a book.
3—Moderate	Fatiguing only if prolonged—like carrying a full handbag that seems heavier as the day goes on.
4—Hard	More than moderate at first, and becoming difficult by the time you complete 6 or 7 repetitions. You can make the effort 12 times in good form but need to rest afterward. Think of lifting a 5-pound sack of potatoes or a gallon of water multiple times.
5—Extremely Hard	Requires all your strength, like lifting a piece of heavy furniture that you can lift only once, if at all.

Working Up Gradually

The ultimate goal is to reach an intensity of 4 for each exercise. But whenever you're trying a new strength-training move for the first time, the intensity should be a 3 or less. You need time to perfect your form and let the muscles get used to each set of moves. After a few workout sessions, it's time to increase the intensity to 4.

To go from a lower to a greater intensity is to work through *progressions*. Progressions will be provided for most of the exercises, and everyone should start with the first progression until the form is mastered. And work up from there.

Try to increase progressions every other workout—or every week—for the first couple of months. For instance, if the progression is to increase the amount of weight you lift, increase the weight by one increment, say, going from 5-pound to 6-pound dumbbells. Of course, as you become stronger, that weight will not seem like so much and the intensity will drop below a 4 again. It's at that point that you should proceed to the next progression, and so on. As you progress over time, the intervals at which you do so will become farther and farther apart. Remember, no matter what progression you are at, always perform two sets of 12 repetitions. The number of reps and sets never changes.

You may find that your muscles feel sore after the first few workouts that are a 4 on the intensity scale (a few people get mild soreness the first couple of times regardless of intensity). That's okay. In fact, it's desirable. It's a sign that you are challenging your muscles to an appropriate degree. But the soreness should *not* interfere with your routine activities. If it does, move down one progression for a week or two.

Don't be discouraged if you move through the progressions for some of the exercises faster than for others. Most people start out with some muscles stronger than others, so progressing more quickly with those is bound to happen. Just bear in mind that *all* of your muscle groups will become stronger if you keep at it. As with aerobic exercise, beginning slowly and progressing gradually but consistently is what works over the long run.

Before You Begin

For safety's sake, you'll need to warm up before you strength-train, just as you do with aerobic activity, with three to five minutes of light activity. You can take a brisk walk around the block or just march in place, but do something with your body before you start lifting. Cooldown for strength training will consist of the stretching exercises described in the Flexibility section later in this chapter.

Tempo and Form

With strength training, the timing of each repetition is everything, and that timing is rather slow. You want to make sure it's your muscles that are doing the work—not gravity and not momentum. To that end, a single lift should take about eight seconds: three to raise the weight, a one-second pause, and four to return to the starting position. Then pause again while you take a breath before starting the next rep. *Never rush your strength training.*

After you have finished a set of reps, rest from 30 seconds to a minute before starting the second set. Resting is not wasting time. That short time interval increases blood flow and nutrients to the muscles and washes away metabolic waste.

For each exercise, there is a correct form. That's how you ensure that you're targeting, or isolating, the right muscles. It is important to actually *visualize* these muscles contracting to lift and stretching while returning to the starting position. The best way to work it is *not* to tense up the other muscles in your body as you're tensing the ones meant to be used for the lift. Use the brief pause after lifting to scan your body for tension in areas other than the muscles you're trying to work—and relax them. These are a couple of areas that commonly tense up when people exercise:

Face: Don't furrow or knit your brow. And don't clench your teeth or tighten your jaw.

Shoulders: Don't scrunch your shoulders up toward your ears. Don't push them forward, either, which only serves to round the chest and keep you from taking full, deep breaths. Keep your shoulders down and back—relaxed. That will relieve tension in your neck, too.

Posture: Along with keeping your shoulders relaxed, keep your chin tucked in, your abdominal muscles firm, and your back straight but relaxed (not arched).

Breathe!

Also important is breathing throughout the exercises. *Never hold your breath.* That can raise blood pressure as you lift the weight, reducing the blood flow to your muscles.

Exhale as you lift the weight, and inhale as you lower it. It is counterintuitive to what you might do naturally, but that's the right way to go. Don't worry if you can't get the right rhythm when you first start. Just keep breathing. As you become more comfortable with the whole process, you'll be able to incorporate the breathing rhythm correctly.

We have found that it really helps people new to strength training to count out loud the eight seconds of each rep. That facilitates breathing *and* doing the exercises at the appropriate tempo.

Make It Your Own
If you do the following exercises twice a week, you'll be doing a lot to get your cardiovascular system—and the rest of your body—in great shape. If you do them three times a week, so much the better. But if you've never strength-trained, you might want to start with only one or two exercises and work up from there. Also, you don't have to do it all on two or three days. If you want to spread it out, you can do these moves over six days—three of them on one day, the other three the next, then back to the first three. Just don't do the same strength-training exercises two days in a row. As we said earlier, your muscles need a day of rest to fully recover from a proper workout.

THE TARGETED STRENGTH-TRAINING PROGRAM

The six exercises that form the strength-training portion of the *Strong Women, Strong Hearts* program were designed to have the greatest impact on the largest number of muscles in the body with as few exercises as possible, so as to streamline the process. While all are good for your cardiovascular system, they confer a lot of other benefits as well, which you'll see as you read on.

EXERCISE 1: DIPS ◆

This exercise strengthens your thigh and hip muscles, making it easier to walk and go up and down stairs and hills. It also improves balance and coordination—even your spatial awareness.

Starting position: Stand with good posture, your body facing the banister of a staircase, your left foot on a step and your right foot parallel but
just to the right and off the step. Hold gently on to the banister with your
hands for balance. If you don't have access to a staircase, use a store-bought
step next to a counter. The step needs to be only 6 inches high.

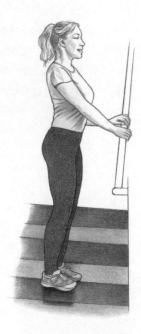 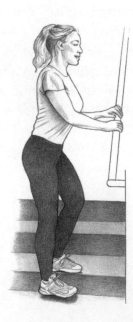

1-2-3-Down: Lower yourself by bending your left leg so that your right foot drops down below the step by about 4 to 5 inches. You will need to bend at the waist. Your buttocks will be back, and your chest high.

Pause for a breath.

1-2-Up: Bring yourself back up to the starting position.

Reps and sets: Repeat the move 12 times on each side—this is one set. Rest for thirty seconds to a minute and then do a second set.

Focal points: Do not let your leading knee go in front of your toes. You will need to engage your abdominal muscles during the movement to stabilize your body.

Progressions
1. Perfect your form by first holding gently on to the banister or counter for balance.
2. Once you can perform this safely, do the exercise without holding.
3. When you can perform this exercise safely without holding on to the banister or counter, hold a 3- to 5-pound dumbbell in each hand, keeping your hands down at your sides at hip level. Continue to maintain proper form in your upper body when using dumbbells. This is a very difficult level; many people never reach this point. Only progress to this level if you feel safe and comfortable.

EXERCISE 2: LUNGE ◆

The lunge targets a large amount of muscle mass in the body, strengthening the thigh, back, and buttocks. It also improves balance and coordination.

Starting position: Stand next to a chair or counter with your feet hip-width apart, knees slightly bent. Lightly hold on to the chair.

1-2-3-Forward: Take a large step forward with your right leg. Land on the heel of your right foot, then roll your foot forward until it is flat on the floor. Keeping your body erect, bend both knees so that your hips drop straight down. Your front thigh should be almost parallel to the floor, and the knee of your back leg should approach the floor. The knee of your forward leg should be over your ankle, not past your toes.

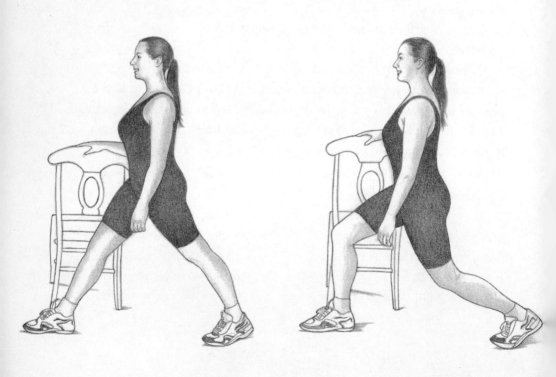

Pause for a breath.

Return: Push back forcefully with the front leg to return to the starting position.

Reps and sets: Alternate legs as you step forward until you have done 12 reps with each leg—this is one set. Rest for thirty seconds to a minute and do a second set.

Focal Points: Do not use the chair to support your weight by leaning on it. Use it only for balance. Maintain posture in the upper body as you descend and ascend, keeping your shoulders and head in line with your hips. Keep the forward leg over the ankle (not in front of it) and in line with the toes. Depending on how tall you are, you may need to adjust the distance between your feet. Distribute your weight between the balls and heels of your feet and equally between the front and back leg. You'll feel the effort in your thighs and back.

Progressions

1. Use the chair for balance and lower with both knees. If you cannot maintain good form when you rise, decrease the distance of your descent. Increase the intensity as you get stronger by dropping down closer to the floor and increasing the distance between your legs.

2. When you are stronger and have more stability and the intensity level drops below a 4, increase the intensity by not using the chair for balance.

3. When you can perform this exercise without using your hand for balance and the intensity drops below a 4, hold a 3- to 5-pound dumbbell in each hand while you do the exercise. Progress to 8 pounds, 10 pounds, and 12 pounds as you get stronger. This is a very difficult level; many people never reach this point. Progress to this level only if you feel safe and comfortable.

EXERCISE 3: OVERHEAD PRESS ◆

The overhead press feels more difficult and more uncomfortable for many women than a lot of other strength-training moves—at least at first. This is because the muscles needed to perform the exercise—the triceps in the upper arms and the deltoids in the shoulders—are often fairly weak. In addition, women tend not to have flexibility in their shoulder muscles, which this exercise also targets. But the benefits make this an exercise worth sticking with. Strengthening the triceps and shoulder muscles *and* the upper back muscles allows for better movements over your head, such as placing a heavy suitcase in the overhead luggage compartment.

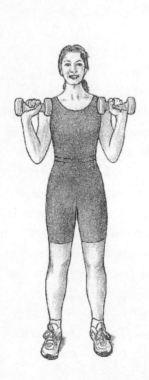
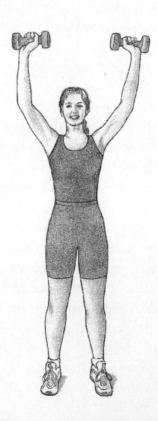

Starting position: You may do this exercise standing or seated in a chair. Your back should be straight, with your head in line with your spine. Hold the dumbbells with palms facing out, shoulder-width apart or slightly more, at a level with your shoulders. Your thumbs will be pointing toward your neck. The dumbbells will be parallel to the floor. Relax your shoulders down your back.

1-2-Up: Press the weights up over your head in a straight line. Do not lock your elbows. Your arms will be above your head and just slightly in front of the plane of your body.

Pause for one second, relaxing your shoulders.

1-2-3-Down: Lower the weights to the starting position.

Reps and sets: Repeat the move 12 times—this is one set. Rest for about thirty seconds to a minute and then do a second set.

Focal points: Keep your upper trunk still during the movement. Initiate the movement in the shoulders. Do not arch your back. The weight is too heavy if you cannot lift it over your head without arching your back. Visualize your shoulders traveling down as you press up. When holding the weights, keep your wrists neutral with your hands fully closed around the dumbbells. Avoid letting the weights bring your wrists too far back or too far forward.

Progressions
1. Start with a 3-pound weight in each hand.
2. As you become stronger and the intensity level decreases below a 4, increase the weight of the dumbbells by 1- to 3-pound increments per workout to reach a 4 on the intensity scale.

Modifications: If you have any shoulder or elbow pain, try rotating your palms toward your neck for the starting position, and maintain this position throughout the lift. Also try keeping your hands shoulder-width apart and no farther.

EXERCISE 4: BICEPS CURL ◆

The biceps are the muscles in the front of your upper arm, and they get a lot of use, as you'll see when you strengthen them. A basket of laundry, a child, a bag of groceries—they'll all be easier to lift as your biceps get stronger. Do not be concerned that you will end up with huge bicep bulges. This exercise, like all other strength-training moves, firms and tones you and makes you feel more confident about wearing a sleeveless blouse. It will not make you muscle-bound.

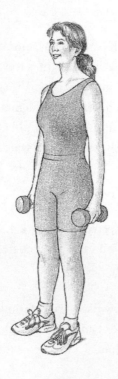 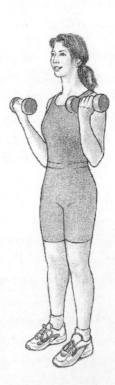

Starting position: Stand with good posture, your feet shoulder-width apart, arms at your sides and your palms facing your thighs, a dumbbell in each hand.

1-2-Up: Slowly rotate your forearms and lift the weights as you bring the dumbbells toward your shoulders. Keep your arms and elbows close to your sides—as if you had a newspaper tucked under each arm. Your palms should be facing your shoulders at the end but not touching them.

Pause for a breath.

1-2-3-Down: Slowly lower your arms to the starting position.

Reps and sets: Repeat the move 12 times—this is one set. Rest for thirty seconds to a minute and then do a second set.

Focal points: Don't let your upper arms or elbows move away from the sides of your body, and keep your wrists straight throughout the move. Hold the dumbbells securely, but don't clench your fists around them.

Progressions

1. Start with a 3-pound weight in each hand.
2. As you become stronger and the intensity level decreases below a 4, increase the weight of the dumbbells by 1- to 3-pound increments per workout to reach a 4 on the intensity scale.

EXERCISE 5: BACK EXTENSION ◆

This exercise strengthens the muscles in your back and buttocks, relieving stress you may feel in your lumbar region, or lower back. It will make activities such as raking leaves, shoveling snow, and vacuuming easier.

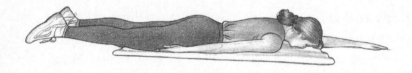

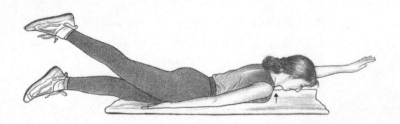

Starting position: Lie facedown with your forehead resting on the floor, legs stretched back, toes pointing back. Extend your left arm straight overhead so that it aligns with your body. Keep your other arm at your side. Tuck your tailbone under you slightly (same as pushing your pubic bone into the floor).

1-2-Up: As you inhale, slowly lift your left arm and right leg off the ground. Keep your arm and leg at the same level. As you lift your arm, your upper back, head, and neck will rise, too. Keep your head, neck, and back in alignment.

Hold the position for three to five seconds.

1-2-3-Down: Exhale as you lower back to the ground.

Sets and reps: Repeat the move 12 times on each side—this is one set. Rest for thirty seconds to a minute and then do a second set.

Focal points: Think of extending up rather than crunching through the lower back. Keep your shoulders back and your chest broadening as you rise and lower down. Keep your head in alignment with your arm; don't overarch your head and neck up. Feel the move throughout your entire back and down into your upper thighs.

EXERCISE 6: ABDOMINAL CURL ◆

Abdominal curls are the *yang* to the back extension's *ying*. They make
your abs tighter and complement your stronger back muscles, thus
improving overall posture. Incidentally, strengthening the abdominal muscles literally tucks in your tummy—*without* the discomfort
of a girdle.

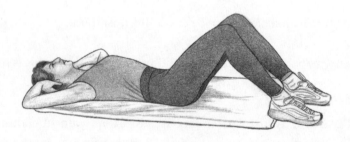

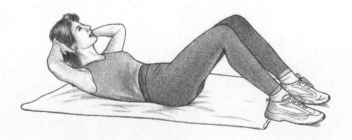

Starting position: Lie faceup, bending your knees but keeping your feet flat on the floor. Make sure your heels are one to two feet from your backside. Interlock your fingers behind the back of your head. This will help to support both your head and your neck as you go through the motion.

1-2-Up: Lift your head and shoulders off the ground by *slowly* contracting your abdominal muscles. You need to bring your back only 3 to 5 inches off the floor. Your chin should be in the neutral position, slightly tucked in but not touching your chest.

Pause for a breath.

1-2-3-Down: Slowly return to the starting position.

Reps and sets: Repeat the move 12 times—this is one set. Rest for thirty seconds to a minute and then do a second set.

Focal Points: When you raise your head, don't pull down with your hands. And don't keep it bent too far forward toward your chest. If your fist fits comfortably between your chin and upper chest, you're doing it right. Also, check for tension—and relax. Think of your stomach as a sponge that is being squeezed. This will help you isolate the right muscles.

THE FLEXIBILITY COMPONENT

The goal of aerobic exercise is to push the heart and the rest of the cardio-vascular system. The goal of strength training is to work the muscles in order for them to adapt and get stronger and also to be more metabolically active. The goal of flexibility is to stretch your muscles, tendons, and ligaments so they become more supple and resistant to injury. You need to exceed your current range of motion for the body to respond and increase that range.

While you'll feel the effects of strength training within two weeks, flexibility comes with time; gains are made in quarter- and half-inch increments. But they'll eventually lead to greater freedom of movement, not to mention fewer aches and pains and a reduced risk of injury.

Before You Begin

Never stretch without being warmed up. You don't want to "snap" your "rubber bands" before you've "loosened" them. But that shouldn't be a problem because you'll be doing your stretching at the end of aerobic and strength-training workouts. (Women who start to do even more athletic training—training for running races or competing in triathlons—need to stretch *before* exercising, too, to minimize overuse injuries.)

Note that a stretch may produce some discomfort, at least at first, but it should never be painful. Use common sense. If your muscle quivers, or if pain persists, you've stretched too much.

Perform each stretch twice. The movements should be slow and deliberate—and then static (not bouncing) for a period of time when you reach your stretching endpoint (the point at which you feel tight but not in pain).

Try to stretch for at least twenty seconds. That's the *minimum* amount you'll need to see gain. Stretching for thirty seconds to a minute is *optimal*.

It's a good idea to stretch every single day—even on those days you do no other exercises. The greatest increases in flexibility come with stretching every day.

HAMSTRING STRETCH ◆

Stand with your feet hip-width apart, knees slightly bent. Do not lock your knees. Pull your tailbone underneath you slightly. Bend forward from the hips and place your outstretched hands on a chair (or a table if the chair is too low). Keep your neck in line with your spine. Center your hips over your ankles. You will feel a stronger stretch in the back of the thighs when you do this. Only bend down as far as you can while maintaining a straight back. You will benefit more by doing this stretch properly but not going down as far, and you will avoid injuring your back. Complete the stretch two times for twenty seconds. When you are ready, increase the time to thirty seconds or more.

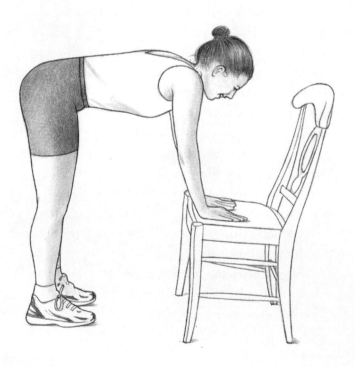

CROSSOVER FOR BUTTOCKS AND HIPS ◆

Lie on your back on the floor with your legs extended. Stretch your left arm out in line with your shoulder. Grasp the outside of your left knee or thigh with your right hand. Inhale, and as you exhale pull your left knee across your body toward the floor. Keep your shoulders and head on the floor. Pull your left leg across your body until you feel the stretch in the outside of your left hip. You may also feel it on the left side of your trunk. Do the same stretch on your right side for the right hip and buttock. Complete the stretch two times for twenty seconds on both sides. When you are ready, increase the time to thirty seconds or more.

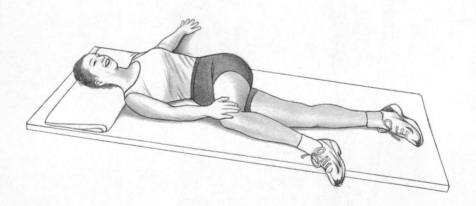

QUADRICEPS STRETCH ◆

Stand behind a chair. Bend your left knee, bring your heel toward your
buttocks, and grasp your foot with your left hand. Pull your heel toward
your buttocks. Do not arch your lower back to get your heel closer. Keep
your knee in line with your hip; do not pull it out, in, forward, or back.
Keep the knee of your right leg bent slightly throughout the move to avoid
straining it. Complete the stretch two times for twenty seconds on both
sides. When you are ready, increase the time to thirty seconds or more. If
you are unable to grasp your foot because you are not yet flexible enough,
place your lower leg on a second chair behind you.

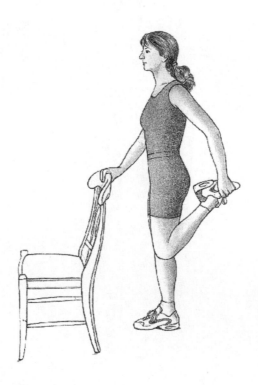

SHOULDER STRETCH ◆

Stand with your feet hip-width apart, knees slightly bent. Relax your shoulders down and back, and keep your head in line with your spine. Interlock your fingers, turn your palms out, and stretch your arms forward. (If you can't turn your wrists enough to interlock your fingers, bend your wrists back as far as they will go and touch the fingertips of your two hands together.) Lift them up toward your head, keeping your shoulders down and back. Keep raising your arms until you feel a stretch in your shoulders.

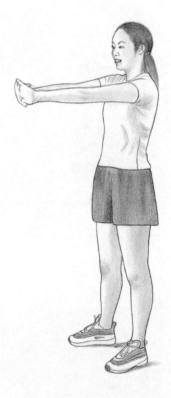

As you lift, do not arch your lower back or drop your head forward. Relax and breathe throughout the stretch. The maximum endpoint is with your arms straight above your shoulders, elbows next to your ears. Keep turning your palms away from you. You will also feel this stretch in the forearms. It does not matter how far you raise your arms, just that the posture is correct and you feel a stretch. Complete the stretch two times, twenty seconds each time. When you are ready, increase the time to thirty seconds or more.

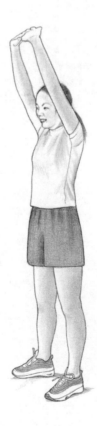

KEEPING TRACK

The best way to ensure that you do the appropriate amount of exercise is to keep a log. Research has shown over and over again that people who keep records of the exercises they do (and the meals and snacks they eat) are the ones most likely to stick to their plan. It forces you to be accountable to yourself. Write in your log, and it "talks back" to you, letting you see where you've kept up and where you've lapsed and need to redouble your efforts.

You can use Miriam's *Strong Women's Journal* or the exercise log below. Simply make multiple copies and keep them in a folder.

GENERAL ACTIVITY Sports games, leisure play, commuting, errands, climbing the stairs, work around the house or garden Goal: as often as you can		
DAY	ACTIVITY	TIME
PLANNED AEROBIC ACTIVITY Goal: 3 to 6 times per week, 30 minutes or more per session		
DAY	ACTIVITY	TIME

STRENGTH TRAINING Goal: 2 to 3 times per week			
EXERCISE 2 SETS/12 REPS	DAY: POUNDS OR "√"	DAY: POUNDS OR "√"	DAY: POUNDS OR "√"
Dips			
Lunges			
Biceps Curl			
Overhead Press			
Abdominal Curl			
Back Extension			
FLEXIBILITY Goal: After each exercise session			
STRETCHES	"√"	"√"	"√"
Hamstring			
Crossover			
Quadriceps			
Shoulders			

STEPS PER DAY (IF YOU USE A PEDOMETER)

Monday	Tuesday	Wednesday	Thursday	Friday	Saturday	Sunday
___	___	___	___	___	___	___

WHAT'S NEXT?

While there's nothing like an exercise routine to ground you, the repetitiveness can become "stale" after a while, which can make the program difficult to stick to.

Feel free to vary the types of exercises you do. Even if you keep doing the same activities, such as brisk walking, some people enjoy finding new places to walk. The visual stimulation of looking at new things could be enough to keep you going. Or you could cross-train: walk one day, swim another, and bike another.

When it comes to strength training, the exercises here certainly cover the gamut of what your body needs, but they are by no means the only ones. We encourage you to vary your strength-training program. Check out one of Miriam's other books; join a fitness center where you can work out on machines; hire a personal trainer for a few sessions to freshen up your routine. You can also learn several different exercise routines by going to www.strongwomen.com or getting some help at a health club. Even if you don't belong to a gym, many of them let you buy a day pass, and you can get strength-training tips from certified trainers on staff.

Helen knows well the value of varying your routine. Along with using a treadmill at the Y (plus resistance machines), she enjoys hiking, bicycling, and, during the winter, cross-country skiing. She actually *looks forward* to exercising. "I don't even think about the fact that I'm protecting my heart as I go," she says. "I just like what I'm doing and I love how I feel when I finish a session."

CHAPTER 7

Ten Tough Strategies for Weight Loss— That Work!

◆

I had been overweight my entire life, even as a child. The only time I wasn't overweight was when I was born. Four years ago, I decided it was time to take charge of my health. I was 268 pounds and a size 24. My blood cholesterol was undeniably high—227; my blood pressure, in the hypertensive range—140/82. Also contributing to my decision: the horrifying experience of having to get off a ride at an amusement park because the bar wouldn't lock over me.

I knew I needed a two-pronged approach: I had to eat properly, and I had to exercise.

I really had to change the way I ate. If you look at my dinner plate now, it's going to be two helpings of vegetables and maybe a potato and some type of protein. Before, it was a huge piece of meat, a huge baked potato, and a small helping of one type of vegetable.

Also, fruit has become my major snack now. Once in a while I have a fat-free pudding or popcorn with just a little bit of spray butter. Before, it was a cookie or cake or candy.

As far as exercise, I started out slowly, but I kept at it.

Nine months into the whole thing, I had lost 60 pounds and joined a gym. Two years after I started, I had lost 125 pounds. I now weigh 143 pounds and wear a size 6. I have maintained this weight for two and a half years. My cholesterol is 169; my blood pressure, 118/76—normal. Not only have I improved my heart health, I have also lost my migraine headaches, my stomach problems, my foot aches, and my backaches. I cannot even begin to describe the feeling of being healthy after all those years.

—Deanne

Two-thirds of all women in the United States are either overweight or obese. That raises the risk for heart disease sevenfold. Weight management is critical. But as with other lifestyle changes, there's no one right way to do it. Deanne, for instance, says she was "a junk-food junkie" and had to initiate changes by substituting more healthful, lower-calorie foods for less nutritious, high-calorie choices. She also says she had to teach herself about portion sizes, remarking that "it was nothing to eat half a box of pasta" before she began to lose weight. Furthermore, she had to begin asking herself many times throughout the day, "Am I really hungry?" If the answer was no, she'd take a few minutes to walk away from the food she wanted to let the wave, or craving, pass. In other words, she made the effort her own, separating her larger goal into various smaller components that she could keep chipping away at.

Her strategy couldn't have been more on the mark. For weight loss, breaking down the goal into simple rules that you can keep track of as you go along makes it much easier. After all, you can't wake up one day and somehow be thinner "cold turkey," the way you can give up cigarettes.

That's where this chapter comes in. We have identified the ten most important guidelines for weight loss—the ones that really make a difference if followed by women who want to finally reach their goal of losing weight to become healthier. That said, however, these guidelines, while tough, are flexible enough that they can be adapted to any lifestyle. They will also help women who are currently at a healthy weight *maintain* that weight as they get older. Indeed, Deanne incorporates many of them to remain at the healthy weight she worked so hard to achieve.

Unfortunately, women who are currently at a healthy weight are in the minority. As we said before, more than 60 percent of all women in the United States are either overweight or out-and-out obese. And the extra weight is substantially increasing their risk for heart disease, so for the sake of their health, it's important that they try to take off some of it. By the same token, many who are not overweight have to work hard to keep creeping pounds at bay. Especially after major life changes, such as getting married, having a baby, getting a divorce, losing a spouse, or after menopause, pounds have a sneaky way of showing up—and raising blood cholesterol, blood pressure, and blood sugar, which in turn raise heart disease risk.

It is by no means necessary to be stick thin to get your risk for heart disease as low as possible. For instance, a woman who is five feet four inches tall and weighs 144 pounds is at a healthy weight. Furthermore, in many women who weigh substantially more than is good for them, losing even just 10 or 20 pounds is enough to significantly reduce blood pressure, blood cholesterol, and blood sugar levels—sometimes to the point that women taking medication no longer need it, or can at least have their dose reduced.

What Do You Have to Lose?

How overweight are you? Twenty pounds? Fifty pounds? More? How did you decide? A lot of women go by the weight they were in high school, or the weight they'd need to be to fit into a certain size. We are constantly amazed when we talk to women about the "creative" ways in which they come up with the amount of weight they need to lose. For instance: "When I was twenty-one, I weighed 115 pounds. Now I'm fifty-seven, have gone through menopause, and have had three children, but 115 is really the weight that worked for me. Yes, I know I weigh 180 now, but that is where I want to be."

That's not realistic. Healthy weight is not a wish; it is a scientific number. Actually, there is more than just the number on the scale that says whether you're at a healthy weight. A number that scientists often use is called your body mass index, or BMI, which is a given weight for a given height.

In the scientific community, a healthy BMI is anything between 19 and 24. Overweight is a BMI of 25 through 29, and obese is 30 or more. What is *your* BMI? To find out, you need to measure your height and get an accurate body weight.

Measure those two numbers in the morning with no clothes or shoes on. Then look for your height at the left side of the table. Go across the column until you get to the number you weigh on the scale, and look at the top of the column to see what BMI your weight corresponds to.

Body Mass Index

1. Read down the first column to locate your height.
2. Read across that row and locate your weight.
3. Read the heading on top of the column—that's your BMI.

UNDERWEIGHT BMI under 19		HEALTHY WEIGHT BMI 19–25							OVERWEIGHT BMI 26–29			
HEIGHT (inches)	18 or less	19	20	21	22	23	24	25	26	27	28	29
58	86	91	96	100	105	110	115	119	124	129	134	138
59	89	94	99	104	109	114	119	124	128	133	138	143
60	92	97	102	107	112	118	123	128	133	138	143	148
61	95	100	106	111	116	122	127	132	137	143	148	153
62	98	104	109	115	120	126	131	136	142	147	153	158
63	101	107	113	118	124	130	135	141	146	152	158	163
64	105	110	116	122	128	134	140	145	151	157	163	169
65	108	114	120	126	132	138	144	150	156	162	168	174
66	111	118	124	130	136	142	148	155	161	167	173	179
67	115	121	127	134	140	146	153	159	166	172	178	185
68	118	125	131	138	144	151	158	164	171	177	184	190
69	122	128	135	142	149	155	162	169	176	182	189	196
70	125	132	139	146	153	160	167	174	181	188	195	202
71	129	136	143	150	157	165	172	179	186	193	200	208
72	132	140	147	154	162	169	177	184	191	199	206	213

Very Overweight BMI 30–39										Extremely Overweight
30	31	32	33	34	35	36	37	38	39	40 or more
143	148	153	158	162	167	172	177	181	186	191+
148	153	158	163	168	173	178	183	188	193	198+
153	158	163	168	174	179	184	189	194	199	204+
158	164	169	174	180	185	190	195	201	206	211+
164	169	175	180	186	191	196	202	207	213	218+
169	175	180	186	191	197	203	208	214	220	225+
174	180	186	192	197	204	209	215	221	227	232+
180	186	192	198	204	210	216	222	228	234	240+
186	192	198	204	210	216	223	229	235	241	247+
191	198	204	211	217	223	230	236	242	249	255+
197	203	210	216	223	230	236	243	249	256	262+
203	209	216	223	230	236	243	250	257	263	270+
209	216	223	229	236	243	250	257	264	271	278+
215	222	229	236	243	250	257	265	272	279	286+
221	228	235	242	250	258	265	272	279	287	294+

We suggest you set small goals—one unit of BMI at a time, which is the equivalent of about 5 pounds (unless you're on the tall side, in which case a single BMI unit can be 6 or 7 pounds). If you're obese, reducing by one BMI unit at a time will slowly but surely get you into the overweight zone. If you're overweight, it will move you slowly toward healthy weight.

For those women who *are* at a healthy weight but have high cholesterol or high blood pressure because over the years they have gone from a BMI of 22 to a BMI of 24, dropping down one or two BMI units will likely lower their risk factors.

Try not to focus simply on weight and BMI by themselves. Focus instead on the *behaviors* we delineate in this chapter, which will help you get to your goal weight.

Of course, as many of you know firsthand, losing weight and keeping it off over the long term is not a snap, helpful guidelines notwithstanding. And, unlike so many diet books that promise you'll never go hungry if you just eat low-carbohydrate or high-protein foods or follow some other gimmick, we are not going to pretend that it is. Because the truth of the matter is that you probably *will* experience some hunger or feelings of deprivation, at least at first, since **the only way you can make real headway in a weight-loss effort is to eat fewer calories than you are used to.** It's perhaps the most difficult health behavior task you'll ever need to engage in. A colleague of ours who had to lose some weight to bring down her blood cholesterol says the first few days in particular were rough, in part because she felt hungry and in part because she was having to reevaluate the way she had always approached food.

THE TEN STRATEGIES FOR EFFECTIVE WEIGHT LOSS

The following ten strategies really *will* make the going a little easier. There are no tricks here, but there *is* a certain alchemy that can be achieved by bringing all the elements of these guidelines together in one effort. That is, while the guidelines are simple on the face of it, their sum is very powerful. Incorporate them into your lifestyle, and you will find it hard *not* to lose excess weight.

Indeed, many of them are put to use by people enrolled in the National Weight Loss Registry. To join the registry, which is maintained by researchers at Brown University and now includes thousands of names, you have to have lost at least 30 pounds and have kept off the weight for at least one year. But the average registrant has lost about *60* pounds and maintained the loss for roughly *five* years!

The ten strategies are divided along two general lines. There are rules about your eating *behaviors* and *mind-set,* and rules related specifically to the *foods* you eat and the *calories* you expend in physical activity.

1. Believe You Can Lose Weight, and Commit to Making the Necessary Changes in Your Diet.

Sounds like fluff, right? Believe you can lose the weight, and you will. Well, the evidence shows that you really do have to turn on a "belief" switch in your head. In the mid-1990s, researchers at the University of Maryland tracked more than fifty women who were following a diet and exercise program for almost a year. Before the program began, the women were asked whether they thought they'd lose weight. A little more than half—the believers—said yes. The rest expected to fail. Nine months later, those who had trusted in their ability to lose weight at the beginning lost 30 percent more weight than those who didn't have much hope for themselves.

Why is believing in yourself so crucial? It helps strengthen your commitment to a task that's going to take a considerable amount of mental and emotional energy, a task that may very well go two steps forward, one step backward. After all, you're going to veer from your plan *sometimes,* and it's at those times most of all that you need to have faith in yourself to be able to get right back on track rather than tell yourself you're a failure who can't stick to anything. That way, a candy bar, for instance, remains what it is—a single candy bar rather than "proof" that you have no willpower. Another way of putting it: Having faith in your ability to commit to lifestyle changes that will lead to weight loss will help you stay with it for the long haul. Deanne knows this firsthand. "There were many times that I would slip," she says. "But I made sure I bounced right back and didn't beat myself up about it."

2. Write Down Every Single Thing You Eat.

Consider the research. In one weight-loss study conducted in California, researchers asked half the participants to write down everything they ate.

There was no counseling on *what* foods to eat, *how much* to eat, *when* to eat, etc. The upshot: those who kept food diaries lost more weight. In another study, investigators found that the best predictor for shedding pounds was not exercise intensity or body weight or anything else that typically goes with dieting. It was whether or not people kept a food journal.

What is it about writing down all the foods (and beverages) they eat that helps people stick to their diets? One thing is that it makes it harder to rationalize going overboard. Once you put the foods you eat "outside of yourself" and onto the page, you can't convince yourself that you "really didn't eat that much." It's all there, right in front of you—whether you took seconds, nibbled on something in the car and so on.

But perhaps even more important, writing down your foods keeps the weight-loss effort front and center at all times. You can't just eat and forget about it. You have to *reckon* with your food choices.

Writing it down also increases commitment and motivation. There's nothing like seeing something in black and white to keep from veering off track. At the same time, seeing that you've made good food choices ratchets up resolve—you're less inclined to mess up the hard work you've already done.

To get the most out of this, *always jot down when you eat as well as under what circumstances. You'll pick up eating patterns you may never have realized.* For instance, perhaps you'll discover that you tend to overeat just before or after late-afternoon work meetings. Maybe you'll find you eat much more than you thought while standing at the kitchen counter after clearing the dinner dishes. Once you begin to pick up your patterns, you can begin to work through solutions for *breaking* them. It could be as simple as reminding yourself that once you leave the table, dinner is over and that a couple of bites here and there could add up to 100 calories (10 pounds in a year's time).

We are so convinced of the value of writing down all the foods you eat that Miriam's book, *The Strong Women's Journal,* makes it easy to record every single day's food choices.

3. Commit to Breakfast.

Both of us are big believers in breakfast. As we previously illustrated, it's a meal at which it's easy to get things lacking in the American diet: calcium (from low- or nonfat yogurt, milk, or cheese); fruit (on top of cereal or mixed into yogurt); and whole grains (in the cereal itself or a slice of whole-wheat toast). Also, if you start the day off with a nutritious breakfast, you'll be less inclined to play fast and loose with your weight-loss effort later in the day. People tend to build on their positive acts. One step toward weight control leads to the next.

But now there's another reason to make sure to eat breakfast as part of a weight-loss plan. Research out of the University of Texas at El Paso analyzed seven days' worth of diet diaries kept by almost 900 women and men and found that eating a hearty meal earlier in the day proved more satiating than the same number of calories eaten later on and thereby blunted overall calorie consumption. In other words, eating a substantial breakfast may work *biologically* to keep you from eating less after nightfall.

The numbers are not hard and fast and are going to be different for different people, but the gist is as follows. Say you consume only 150 calories at breakfast—a slice of toast with margarine and a cup of coffee with milk. You might end up totaling 2,000 calories for the entire day. But if you eat 300 to 400 calories at breakfast—maybe a serving of whole-grain cereal with fresh or frozen berries and a banana with a cup of skim milk, along with coffee—you might eat only 1,800 calories by the time the day is over.

Why do people seem to feel more sated by food eaten earlier in the day? The biological mechanism hasn't been worked out, but it could be that the body is set to certain diurnal rhythms that don't jibe with the current human lifestyle. That is, maybe our mechanism for feeling full is in full swing in the morning, when we need enough calories to get through the day. But then it shuts off when the sun goes down because throughout most of our evolutionary history, people pretty much went to sleep at nightfall and therefore didn't need to feel sated to conduct more activity.

Of course, today, with artificial light created by electricity, people remain active long into the evening, with lots of opportunities to eat and not feel sated. Indeed, in the Texas research, as the day wore on, the intervals between eating episodes lessened—regardless of the number of calories eaten. Think of it in terms of your own lifestyle. It might be hours between breakfast and lunch but a relatively short time between a rather heavy dinner and a high-calorie snack between dinner and bedtime.

We don't want to suggest that eating too little at breakfast is the only reason people overeat at night. It's not. There's television watching, boredom, eating to de-stress, and all sorts of other reasons. But since eating a reasonably substantial breakfast can potentially curb the trend and provide a healthful first meal at the same time, along with motivating you to keep on track as you start your day, we wholeheartedly support it.

Breakfast doesn't have to be eaten soon after you wake up. Some people, Alice included, often aren't hungry as soon as they awake and take their breakfast to work with them. Delaying breakfast is okay—as long as it happens!

4. Eat Only at a Table Designated for Dining—Whether It's in Your Kitchen, Dining Room, or Office—*without the TV.*

Thirty years ago, you would never have seen someone eating a bagel on a bus, or wolfing down a slice of pizza while walking along the street, or chomping on drive-through fare in the car. Meals were eaten around a table—without the television on. But with the explosion of cheap, highly palatable convenience foods, people's whole way of eating has changed. And we believe it has contributed to the precipitous rise in body weight seen in recent decades.

When you eat on the run, you tend to eat extremely fast—too fast for your brain to pick up signals of satiety from your stomach. It takes about twenty minutes for the GI tract to inform the brain that you're full. If you're eating really fast because you want to finish a 500-calorie burger or pastry before you reach the entry ramp to a highway, or because you're trying to do twenty things at once and aren't focusing on your food, or because you're in the family room watching TV and not paying attention, you can end up consuming a lot more calories than your body is actually hungry for. If you sit at a table, on the other hand, you're eating *mindfully.* You're focusing on the food, which in itself slows things down.

You're also tasting your food better—slower chewing allows for a fuller gustatory experience, with more flavors and textures perceived. That, too, can cut down on the amount you eat because you feel more satisfied with less.

Eating in a relaxed manner has the same effect. The more you enjoy the dining *experience,* the less you need to get what you need out of it by heaping on more food. And the less you'll hurriedly sneak in a lot of calories without realizing it, say, by tasting too often while cooking, finishing the left-overs in the serving dish, or eating what a small child has left on her or his plate. All of these things tend *not* to happen in calm moments at the table but in those almost imperceptible, stress-filled moments between not wanting to overdo and having overdone it before you have had a chance to reason with yourself.

We cannot emphasize enough how important it is to make sure you eat all meals and snacks in a relaxed manner without a lot of distractions—including the television. There is a very strong relationship between the amount of TV someone watches and the degree to which she is overweight.

As busy as we both are, we make a point of dining this way. No one ever eats away from the table in either of our houses except for those rare times when someone is sick in bed and is served soup upstairs or, for instance, the family is making a special night of it by watching the Super Bowl and enjoying some popcorn in front of the television. Also, we try hard to leave work every night before six o'clock no matter how busy we are because we want to get home and have dinner with our families.

Those times when meals become haphazard, all bets are off. The eating gets less healthful, the calories are piled on willy-nilly because it's hard to keep track when you're scarfing down foods on the go, and all enjoyment of food—which is even more important when you're trying to eat less of it—goes out the window.

Granted, sitting down to meals is not always easy for a family to negotiate. A teenager has swim practice after school, for instance, or somebody comes home late from work several times a week. But the more you can create a pattern for eating together when it *is* possible, the better attention to calories you are going to be able to pay.

5. Set a Kitchen-Closed Time—and Stick to It.

In a study in Sweden, investigators found that obese women tended to eat the same number of calories as healthy weight women throughout most of the day, yet ate significantly more calories from eight in the evening until midnight.

Perhaps you recognize yourself as an evening eater. A lot of people are, and for a lot of reasons—boredom, TV food ads, and the list goes on. If you make a pact with yourself not to eat after dinner, you will save hundreds of calories a day. Evening is prime time for ice cream, chocolate, chips and nuts, all of which can be gobbled in minutes.

People's kitchen-closed times will vary. Some people don't get home from work until late. That is okay. The point is to stop dinner from becoming the beginning of an eating activity that continues until you go to bed.

6. Be Extra Vigilant When You Haven't Prepared the Food Yourself.

Both of us believe firmly that preparing your own meals as often as possible is one of the best ways to limit calories and improve your diet. When you cook the meal, you control what, and how much, you're eating. But the reality is that many women are already maxed out time-wise and simply have to rely, at least in part, on restaurant food, takeout food, and prepared supermarket foods. Indeed, more than half of us eat at least one meal away from home on any given day, according to a government survey known as "What We Eat in America."

That's why it's so important to be aware that food prepared outside your own kitchen tends to be higher in calories than food you make yourself and that it's important to eat such food with special attention to portion size. A study conducted by some of our colleagues at Tufts makes the point all too well. The researchers looked at the frequency with which six dozen women and men visited seven different kinds of restaurants, including those that specialized in fried chicken, burgers, pizza, Chinese or Mexican foods, and fried fish. The more often the subjects ate out, the higher their calorie consumption, and the higher their level of body fatness. It was that simple.

So when you eat out or order in, choose wisely. In a sit-down restaurant, really do ask for at least half the portion to be wrapped up before it's even brought to the table. Or, upon getting something home, immediately put at least half in the fridge for another meal. Don't trust your willpower, which will be in short supply when you're hungry and tired.

And don't be afraid to ask for meals in restaurants exactly as you want them. After all, you're paying for them!

Miriam was in a restaurant in Bellingham, Washington, recently, and the waiter was kind enough to reassure her that if she wanted to double the vegetable and halve the potato, that was fine. You really *can* have it your way, even if the restaurant doesn't have a little jingle to prove it.

Alice knows this from experience, too. When she was staying in a New Hampshire inn recently for a little cross-country ski break, she asked for the kitchen to hold the sauce on her fish, double the vegetables, and hold the scalloped potatoes (which contained cream and butter she didn't want). She was not perceived as difficult. The staff was happy to oblige. If enough of us ask for these types of changes to menus, food will start to be served this way routinely and we won't have to ask anymore.

7. Don't Drink Your Calories.

The calories you drink don't end up making you feel as full as the calories you eat. Researchers at Purdue University in Indiana made the point when they gave people either 400 calories' worth of sugary jelly beans or 400 calories' worth of sugary soda pop. The people given the jelly beans ate fewer calories later in the day to compensate for their jelly bean consumption. The soda drinkers did not.

Researchers suspect that liquids just don't trigger satiety mechanisms in the gastrointestinal tract in the same way that solids do. Whatever the reason, all the calories Americans now consume from beverages are no doubt contributing to the national epidemic of overweight and obesity. Soft drinks are *the* leading source of added sugars in our diets; consumption of carbonated beverages has risen 500 percent since the 1950s! Consumption of many kinds of fruit and fruit-based juices and drinks, none of which has any of the fiber of actual fruit, has increased 280 percent. (And 100 percent fruit juice tends to have as many calories as sweetened juice beverages. Don't be fooled into thinking that juice per se is relatively low in calories.)

Then there are all the newfangled drinks at coffee shops, many of which have more calories than the pastry or doughnuts sold alongside them. A caramel cappuccino has 350 calories; a white chocolate mocha 440.

We believe every calorie you take in should be *felt,* especially when you're trying to make each calorie count because you're cutting back. And since liquid calories are not well perceived by the body, we feel strongly that thirst should be quenched only by water or a cup of nonfat or 1% milk here or there. If diet soft drinks or coffee or tea sweetened with artificial sweetener help you limit calories, use them. We don't *advocate* use of artificial sweeteners. But for some people, they *can* have a place in a reduced-calorie diet.

8. Eat Grains, But Make Them *Whole* Grains.

As pointed out in chapter 5, some people think that carbohydrates have a special tendency to add fat to the body. They don't. In fact, whole-grain carbohydrates can aid a weight-loss effort. In research conducted here at Tufts, one of our colleagues switched people from refined grains to whole grains, with the result that they started complaining immediately that they were being given too much to eat! They were not getting any more calories. But whole grains, unlike refined, contain fiber, which can help fill you up.

The average person eats only one serving of whole grains per day and six to twelve—or more—servings of refined grains. That many servings even of whole grains is too much, certainly for a weight-loss effort. So our advice here is twofold, and while it's simple to say, it takes some planning.

First, while you are actively losing weight, stick only with whole grains. Second, limit whole grains to no more than four to six servings a day. Remember, a serving is a 1-ounce slice of bread, a half cup of brown rice or whole-wheat pasta, or a portion of whole-grain cereal (oatmeal is a whole grain), as listed on the side of the cereal box. (It's okay to eat a whole cup of whole-wheat pasta at once. Just be sure to count it as two servings.)

Eating only whole grains may be more difficult than you think—at first. Only 5 percent of the grain-based foods in the supermarket are whole—and probably less in restaurants. But it will really fuel your weight-loss effort, in no small part because it removes from your eating plan a lot of foods people tend to overdo: regular pasta, cakes and cookies (both made with white flour), oversized bagels (a 5-ounce bagel is the caloric equivalent of five slices of Wonder bread), pretzels, and most crackers.

9. Snack Smart.

We wholeheartedly endorse snacking, as our menus show. It staves off hunger between meals and provides an opportunity to consume essential nutrients.

But a snack is not a 200-calorie energy or candy bar, or a 150-calorie chips. It's an 80-calorie apple or a 120-calorie cup of nonfat yogurt.

How do you get yourself to eat those foods instead of cookies, power bars, and the like? Buy them and not the other stuff—and keep them front and center either in a fruit bowl on the kitchen counter or right in front of the refrigerator on an eye-level shelf; or in your handbag at work so they are readily available. *You* control the nosh choices.

Interestingly, there has been some research associating low- and nonfat dairy foods like yogurt with weight control. Two recent studies have found that in both women and men, a diet rich in low-fat dairy was linked with lower body weight. Other preliminary research has found, similarly, that increased servings of dairy products are associated with lower body *fat*.

Why isn't clear. Most likely, dairy is a marker for eating healthfully in general. Another speculation is that dairy may stimulate weight loss by increasing fat metabolism. The effect, if there indeed is one, is modest. We are not at all pretending that if you just add dairy foods to your diet, you'll magically lose a lot of extra weight. But since two to three servings of dairy foods are needed each day for general good health anyway, snacks are a good place to incorporate them. Just be sure they're low in fat—and sugar. A lot of yogurts are loaded with sugar, which can increase calories considerably.

Also, *plan ahead*. Make sure to always have fresh fruit and dairy at home, or bring it to the office. When the 4:30 afternoon lull hits, you want to have the right snack on hand.

10. Move Your Body.

It's not impossible to lose weight without exercise, but it's certainly difficult—and not good for you, either. Almost every single person in the National Weight Control Registry exercises regularly, by which we mean almost every day. They know intuitively what a National Institutes of Health Task Force on Obesity stated several years ago. When you're trying to lose weight, 75 percent of the calorie deficit comes from eating less food—and 25 percent comes from burning more calories through increased physical activity. The weight-loss registrants have also learned what studies keep showing: nine in ten weight losers who do not exercise gain the weight back.

Walking is the most convenient form of exercise. A 150-pound woman will burn 80 to 100 calories for each mile she walks. Of course, even walking just one mile might seem daunting to someone who needs to lose a substantial amount of weight but hasn't exercised in years—or perhaps ever. Likewise, as we discussed in chapter 6, lifting weights to rev up metabolism could also be difficult for someone who has never strength-trained.

Don't take our word for it; take Deanne's. Exercising "wasn't easy," she comments. "I remember the early days of lifting cans of baked beans and one-liter bottles of water. I soon progressed to five- and ten-pound weights and more and more walking on the treadmill. A year and a half after starting, I even discovered that I liked running. I had tried many times over the years to run but always hated it. I guess I finally hit a weight at which it became enjoyable."

SLOW AND STEADY WINS THE RACE

You may not want to tackle all ten of our strategies all at once. That's okay. But if you are going to make a serious attempt at losing weight, you are going to need to tackle most of them or else find your own healthy way to lose the pounds. In the end you need to eat less and move more. Right now, think about which strategies you are going to adopt first and how you are going to do so.

We have found with many women that each step is a building block that propels them on to others. Start small, as Deanne did, and before long you'll have an arsenal of weight-loss approaches that you're employing to make the most of your weight-loss efforts as quickly as possible.

But do start. If you are overweight, you simply are not going to shed any excess pounds without making some serious adjustments to your daily habits—that could take getting used to. If you wait until you feel "just right" about it, you could go your whole life weighing more than you should. There will always be something getting in your way, so you might as well jump in *now*—not tomorrow morning—and get the ball rolling. Make the switch in your brain to one of commitment and belief. It won't feel as difficult after a week or two of building the changes into your routine.

Says Deanne, "After a while, losing weight becomes a self-fulfilling thing.

The more you lose, the easier it gets to keep it up. In my case, my self-esteem and confidence were soaring as my pants size was dropping.

"At some point every day I still have to make a decision not to eat something that's not good for me or that I'm not hungry for. There's no day that goes by where I don't get challenged. But I've learned to listen to my body. I make smarter choices. It really has gotten easier."

CHAPTER 8

Relaxing, Taking a Deep Breath, and Other Approaches

❖

Your heart "races" or "pounds" from stress or anger. "Skips a beat" when you feel afraid. "Sinks" when you're low or depressed. Even if you've never made the connection consciously, the fact that our emotions and our hearts are inextricably interwoven is so well intuited that the notion is embedded in our very language.

The Bible itself makes reference to it. When Jacob heard that his son, Joseph, had been alive the entire twenty-two years he had been missing in Egypt, his heart "fell" from the shock. Biblical scholars have interpreted it to mean that he suffered a heart attack.

Today, a growing body of research is beginning to confirm scientifically what people have always known "in their hearts": Stress, whether experienced as anxiety, depression, or some other emotion, affects cardiovascular health. A lot of the evidence centers around the impact of emotional health in heart disease that has already been diagnosed. For instance, it has been shown that depression increases the risk for a second heart attack. But there's more and more evidence that stress, anguish, and related mental states play a role in the *development* of heart disease as well.

STRESS AND HOSTILITY'S DIRECT EFFECT

Stress and its influence on the heart can be hard to quantify, but one telling study conducted in Sweden in the 1990s makes the connection. Researchers there compared city bus drivers to bus drivers in rural areas. What they found was that bus drivers in urban settings were more likely to die from heart disease than other workers in the same geographical area, but rural bus drivers had the same rate of heart disease death as other workers in their locale. As anyone who has ever ridden on a city bus knows, driving one entails *a lot* of stress; thus, the researchers concluded, stress played into urban bus drivers' worse rates of cardiovascular death than those experienced by their rural counterparts.

Several studies have also spotlighted anger, including one from the University of North Carolina. Researchers there gave an anger "test" to some 13,000 people, asking them whether they tended to fly off the handle, say unkind things when angry, or become furious when slowed down by others (think traffic jam or having to reexplain something). The higher they scored, the more likely they were to suffer heart problems down the line. In fact, the most anger-prone people had nearly a threefold greater risk of suffering a heart attack or dying from heart disease than those with a longer fuse.

Another study, conducted at the University of Michigan, showed that hostile people, when asked to relive an angry memory, had larger and longer-lasting rises in blood pressure than others. And a third study, out of California, suggested that hostility starts hurting the heart early in life. Young adults with scores above average on an anger test were more likely than others to have already undergone some calcification in their coronary arteries, which is one of the steps contributing to advanced atherosclerosis.

Along with raising blood pressure and paving the way for the faster development of atherosclerosis, anger is believed to prompt the release of stress hormones such as cortisol and catecholamines. Over the long term, all these stress hormones flooding the system can damage the delicate linings of blood vessels surrounding the heart. They can disrupt the heart's electrical rhythm, too. And they set in motion a process whereby blood platelets become "stickier" and clump together, which may in turn set the stage for a heart attack or stroke.

Not surprisingly, people with a hostile outlook tend to get themselves into angry confrontations more often, which only sets the whole chain of events into action with a consistency that increases the risk for heart problems that much more.

HOW DEPRESSION TAKES ITS TOLL

Some people have characterized depression as anger turned inward. Whether you subscribe to that definition or not, depression, which affects women disproportionately, can be just as bad for the heart as hostility. Research at Montreal's McGill University has found that depressed people have a three to four times higher risk of dying within eighteen months of having a heart attack.

Another study has found that depressed people are more likely to end up with heart disease in the first place. Ten years after a group of women and men took a depression test at a time when all of them were heart disease–free, those whose test scores showed evidence of depression were 70 percent more likely than the others to have suffered a heart attack or developed ischemia or some other form of heart disease.

Why? It could be that people with depression have difficulty following lifestyle recommendations to prevent heart problems. Because of their condition, many times they cannot take proper care of themselves by adhering to a heart-healthy diet or getting adequate exercise. A Johns Hopkins University School of Medicine study has shown, in addition, that heart attack survivors diagnosed with depression are less likely than their nondepressed counterparts to adhere to treatment recommendations meant to reduce their risk for a second cardiac event down the line.

But there's more to it than not taking care of themselves. People with depression also have a lower heart rate variability, meaning their hearts are less adaptable to situations and won't change their "pace" sufficiently when they go, for example, from sitting in a chair to climbing a staircase (refer to the box on page 58).

Furthermore, while depressed people may often seem in low gear, they are actually in a state of high arousal much of the time, just as angry people are. Thus, they release high levels of stress hormones that unduly tax the cardiovascular system. (Depression may look sluggish on the outside but can really be churning up the system from the inside.)

STEPS FOR GAINING EMOTIONAL EQUILIBRIUM

Angry, depressed, or just plain stressed out, you don't have to live with the negative state of mind—and let it keep taking a toll on your heart. There's much you can do, literally, to blunt negative emotions, whether that means stopping to smell the roses or seeing the world a little more rose-colored.

Sometimes it's just a matter of working to see things through a different angle of life's prism. For instance, maybe you have a coworker who always tries to take credit for projects that you have a big hand in bringing forward. Of course it's annoying. But maybe it pays to consider that it might very well make the person look petty to the higher-ups, at least some of whom have to be aware of all your hard work.

Or maybe you often feel stressed because there are frequent delays and interruptions—through no fault of your own—in your already very tightly scheduled day. And those delays make you lose it—you start snapping at your office mates or family. Perhaps the solution is to acknowledge up front that things never run as smoothly as one would like and plan fewer tasks per given amount of time. That may feel like inefficiency, but in the end it could actually be more pragmatic. You get to focus fully on each task at hand, and you don't end up angry and disappointed that you weren't able to get more done.

Sometimes even just acknowledging openly to yourself what's gnawing at you can help to put it into proper perspective. It reminds you that there are more dimensions to life than whatever is so troubling at that very moment.

Along with turning life's frustrations on their ear a little, there are a number of anxiety-reducing practices that millions of people use across the globe to get "centered" and thereby take better care of themselves emotionally—and thereby take better care of their hearts. Check out the ones below to see if any might be right for you.

Meditation (Birkenstocks Not Required)

Many people hear the term "meditation," and they think it means sitting cross-legged on the floor in flowing robes or a loincloth. It doesn't. In fact, it's a rather mechanical process. For instance, in a type of meditation called *transcendental meditation,* you simply sit for twenty minutes twice a day with your eyes closed. During that quiet time, you repeat a mantra—a soothing sound—that allows the mind and body to settle down, so to speak, and "release" stress and hostility. The result is a deep state of restful alertness. That is, the body is at rest, but the mind becomes more wakeful, or lit, from within. That gets the mind and body into balance.

People generally link meditating, or being in a meditative state, with stress reduction. And rightly so. What's less well known is that in some cases, meditation can lower blood pressure as well as drugs can. We believe all types of meditation can have this effect, but the research to date has focused on transcendental meditation, which is why we refer specifically to that type here. In a project involving more than 100 people at California's West Oakland Health Center, those who learned and performed transcendental meditation every day for three months experienced an overall drop in systolic pressure that was greater than the drop in people who simply were counseled on lifestyle changes such as losing excess weight, cutting back on salt, and drinking less alcohol. The meditators' diastolic pressure also dropped more than in the group receiving only lifestyle advice. Comparable reductions in blood pressure achieved with drugs have been linked with substantial reductions in stroke risk and congestive heart failure.

Meditation not only lowers blood pressure, but by reducing stress, it can also help people curb unhealthful behaviors that get in the way of their heart-healthy efforts. Consider that people in the Oakland study who did not meditate did not make any appreciable changes in their lifestyle habits. But the meditation group went from roughly eleven drinks a week to five—which, for women, meant going from too much alcohol to an amount that's consistent with protection against heart disease. That, combined with the stress reduction imparted by meditation, could benefit the heart that much more.

For those who want to try meditation, major cities across the country have local centers, listed in the phone book under "Meditation," that teach this relaxation technique.

Tai Chi

It's now fairly well established that tai chi, an ancient, graceful martial arts form in which slow movements flow one into the other, lowers the body's

Herbs, Roots, and Other Complementary Therapies

Meditation, tai chi, yoga—all of these are effective practices for reducing heart disease risk. But along with *doing* things to ward off heart disease, a lot of women are *taking* substances purported to have heart-helping powers. And those substances are now getting serious scrutiny from the medical community. The National Institutes of Health is currently devoting considerable resources to studying adjunctive therapies that include plant extracts and other naturally occurring compounds.

To date, the evidence of benefit for many of those substances is slim to nonexistent. Until the new research results become available, it is too early to recommend them.

For instance, despite promising results from some early research into garlic's effect on lowering blood cholesterol, eight well-controlled trials have shown no improvement in people taking garlic for six months. More than two dozen studies examining garlic's effect on blood pressure also came up "empty."

It's a similar story for coenzyme Q10, a vitamin-like, fat-soluble substance. Trials examining its effects on heart failure patients have shown no benefits. Neither have trials looking at coenzyme Q10 for treatment of angina or hypertension.

Hawthorne root has been recommended for treatment of heart disease in many herbal medicine books. It has even been approved for heart failure patients in Germany and is marketed as a prescription drug there. But the clinical evidence for hawthorne root is less than astounding. In one look at eight studies with a total of some 600 patients, all of whom had congestive heart failure, the only plus to taking hawthorne root appeared to be an ability to exercise longer on a bicycle test, and even that benefit has not been confirmed.

More important, hawthorne root and other complementary treatments have some potentially serious side effects. Hawthorne root can cause nausea, fatigue, sweating, palpitations, and agitation. Coenzyme

Q10 can potentially interact with other drugs. Other substances that some people take to protect their hearts, such as the herb ginkgo biloba, can interfere with blood coagulation, which could be a very serious problem should you bleed as the result of an accident or have to undergo surgery, where bleeding is an expected part of the procedure.

Furthermore, while as many as 75 percent of Americans take some kind of complementary or alternative substance, as few as 17 percent tell their physicians about it. And that leaves doctors in the dark—and patients at risk for serious interactions between drugs that the doctors prescribe and over-the-counter herbs and other substances that the patients decide to take on their own.

If you want to try an over-the-counter preparation to help your heart, discuss it with your doctor, even if you think he or she will pooh-pooh your decision. What may seem like only trying to avoid a lecture about wasting your money could actually be a way of avoiding the use of your body as a site for a very dangerous science experiment.

level of the stress hormone cortisol. It also lowers blood pressure. In a Johns Hopkins study, a group of people who practiced tai chi lowered their systolic pressure by an average of 7 points—just 1 point less than a separate group who engaged in low-impact aerobic dance. Now new research from some of our colleagues at Tufts, in conjunction with investigators at McGill University, has found that tai chi is associated with improved cardiovascular function in general. That's what they found when they conducted a review of nearly fifty studies on tai chi published over the last twenty years.

The relaxing moves, or poses, of tai chi, which have names like White Crane Spreads Its Wings and Step Up to Seven Stars, emphasize balance, breathing, and body awareness. The aim is always on slow, deep breathing and focusing your energy.

Your local Y or health club probably offers a tai chi class. There are also good tai chi videos that you can practice with at home. (See the Resources section at the back of the book.) Keep in mind that tai chi can be posturally demanding. Thus, if you have balance problems, say, because of a medication you are taking, you should speak with your instructor before signing up so your program can be modified accordingly.

Yoga

While the research regarding yoga's direct effects on heart health is scant, there are many reasons to believe that it has a beneficial effect. It is well accepted that in addition to improving physical fitness, yoga increases the mind's capacity for meditation. And since meditation relieves stress, which thereby helps the heart, it's fair to say that yoga is good for the heart.

Yoga often brings to mind people who contort themselves into pretzel-like poses while seeking spiritual enlightenment. Yet yoga is not just for the superflexible, double-jointed minority. Up to 10 million Americans currently engage in this ancient practice, which originated in India.

There are actually many types of yoga, but the kind most Americans think of is *hatha* yoga, which involves a variety of static postures, or *asanas.* Concentrated breathing exercises, or *pranayamas,* are involved, too.

Your local Y or health club is a good place to try on yoga for size by taking a class. Look for an instructor with several years' experience, and make sure her or his style feels right to you. There is no national standardized credentialing program for yoga instructors, so you need to go with your gut.

Optimism

Optimism may not seem like something you can *do,* like yoga or tai chi. But it actually is possible to cultivate optimism, which can break the cycle of depression and thereby improve heart health. (Yes, optimistic people have less heart disease than pessimists.)

How? By disputing negative thoughts—literally. Let's say the pessimistic thought "I'll never be able to lose weight" keeps running through your mind. Is that factually correct, or just an overreaction? Consider the evidence before you decide. Were there times in the past when you were able to reach a difficult goal? The answer is probably yes.

Also, instead of blaming yourself, as pessimistic thinkers tend to do, go over all the contributing factors to the situation and work through how they might be overcome. Is it really a matter of your not being able to stick with a plan, or is it that you actually stick very well to your plans but simply have many competing commitments right now and are having a hard time finding the emotional energy to fit in one more thing? Answering that question honestly will free you up to begin making some changes toward your goal rather than keep you stuck in the erroneous belief that you're simply not capable.

Pessimists can also brighten their outlook by writing things down. When you put your stress outside of yourself by keeping a journal, it's easier to look at your situation objectively and see where you're being held back rather than just assuming nothing will ever get better and the ball is out of your hands. It's not.

Social Outreach

Social isolation is one of the worst things for stress and depression. It gives negativity every opportunity to fester—and worm its way into your heart, both figuratively and literally. Indeed, research has shown that depressed people who live alone or have little contact with friends and relatives are at greater risk for death after a heart attack than depressed people who have a good social support network. Furthermore, people with only a small network of family and friends have a two- to threefold greater risk for developing heart disease over time than others.

If you have been socially isolated, the thought of "getting out there" may seem overwhelming. One option is to find a walking partner. It fosters friendship without forcing it, and you'll get some exercise, too!

We also suggest volunteer work. It builds a social component into your life without putting the emphasis on socializing per se. That, in turn, assuages anxiety about getting together with other people. Yet it will work to extend your social contacts, put you back "in the loop," and bring your mind to a better place—particularly worthy benefits if you've recently been widowed or divorced and therefore might be at increased risk for social isolation because of depression, or perhaps because you're feeling like "a fifth wheel" around other couples you've always socialized with.

Volunteering opportunities abound. You can work for a political or social cause, serve food in a soup kitchen, mentor young people, and so on. You can also inquire at your local schools, hospital, community center, library, or place of worship to see if volunteers are needed.

Talk It Out

Perhaps the most important key for reducing the mental stress in your life in order to protect your heart is to bring it up to your doctor. The vast majority of stressed and depressed patients never get treatment because they never seek it. And doctors don't ask about it. In fact, if you wait for your physician to ask whether something is bothering you, you may wait forever because most physicians are not trained to talk to patients about their feelings. Yet ironically, the medical community is better equipped than ever to treat depression, anxiety, and hostility.

Indeed, in a small study published several years ago, heart patients on standard diet regimens who also sought and got emotional help— either in the form of group therapy, instruction in relaxation techniques, or stress management training—showed greater reductions in psychological distress. They were also able to lower their blood pressure, heart rate, and blood cholesterol.

Your doctor might refer you to a group therapist or psychologist for one-on-one sessions. A doctor can also discuss with you prescription drugs for depression or anxiety. Sometimes even just expressing to your physician that you have undue stress or depression gets the healing process under way.

Speaking of Your Place of Worship . . .

For hundreds of years, Western medicine has treated the body and the soul separately. But the pendulum appears to be swinging back. More and more medical schools are now offering classes on spirituality and medicine. It's not surprising. In a study of patients who had undergone open-heart surgery, those who reported that they drew strength and comfort from religion appeared to have better outcomes after surgery than those who didn't.

The faithful seem to recover from depression more quickly, too. In a look at almost 100 people who became depressed after a hospital stay, researchers at Duke University found that those who scored high on a test of religious beliefs and experience bounced back faster than others. Other research suggests that religious people are less likely to become depressed in the first place.

Still more research has shown that people who attend services at least once a week—or frequently pray or study the Bible at least once a day—have slightly lower blood pressure than those who aren't as religiously active.

Faith appears to affect health on a number of fronts. One is so-called sin avoidance. Religious people often live relatively healthful lives—no smoking or excessive drinking, for instance. Organized religion also increases one's social circle, which buffers the harmful effects of isolation, stress, anxiety, and depression. And prayer itself can be akin to meditation: The repetition in prayer, such as occurs with going through the Catholic rosary or *davening* (a swaying movement during certain prayers in some forms of Judaism), can be compared to repeating a mantra, and the quiet, contemplative mood can be relaxing and profound.

Of course, you can't just march into a church, synagogue, or mosque and expect your heart to get healthier. Faith is deeply held, and commitment to one's faith has a lot to do with its benefits.

The good news: you don't have to be devout or spiritually inclined to reap many of the benefits. Through meditation, social outreach, volunteering, and plain old good, clean living, you're taking advantage of all the secular advantages religion affords. That is, by availing yourself of the approaches in this chapter, as well as in the chapters on nutrition and exercise, you'll be treating your body like a temple—and giving your heart (and soul) the "nourishment" it needs.

PART 3

Beyond
Lifestyle

Sorting Through the Medication Options

◆

I was so disappointed that despite all my efforts to bring down my blood pressure through lifestyle—giving up alcohol, eating more than five fruits and vegetables a day, going easy on the saltshaker, walking or running five miles three times a week, and strength training twice a week—I still had to go on medication to get it into line. And then the dose had to be doubled because it started to creep up again. But when I told my internist how bad I felt about it, he reminded me that other people in my family got high blood pressure in their thirties and forties, whereas I was able to hold off until I was fifty. "That's really great," he said. "Your preventative lifestyle kept it at bay for much longer." He was right. That made me feel better about it.

—ANNE

When it comes to taking a drug to control the course of a disease, many women fall into one of two camps. One camp holds the position that resorting to a drug means they've failed in their efforts to control the disease on their own; they resist taking the medicine because they feel it would mean they've failed at strong-arming the problem and may even resort to spending a lot of money on unproven over-the-counter preparations. The other camp's perspective is that the drug will "take care of the problem." As long as the pill is popped, they're all set and don't have to pay attention to anything else.

Neither one of those attitudes has any place in heart disease treatment. While lifestyle changes are the first line of defense for decreasing blood cholesterol and blood pressure to reduce the risk for heart attacks and strokes, in no way should you misconstrue a prescription for a drug as license to abandon your efforts to eat a heart-healthy diet and get adequate exercise. Both the National Institutes of Health and the American Heart Association are quite clear that the best outcomes happen to those people who continue to protect their hearts through lifestyle changes as they follow through with a prescription. Reverting to a poor diet and a sedentary way of living—and letting your weight creep up—not only reduces the benefit, it can work against you by making it harder for the drug to do its job. Indeed, we have heard anecdotally that some people have been known to eat their way around a drug, making it difficult to control their blood cholesterol levels even though the drugs to keep down cholesterol are so powerful.

As for those who feel that resorting to a drug means that they couldn't "cut it" and are officially sick, nothing could be further from the truth. Taking the right medication means you're taking advantage of the best twenty-first-century medicine has to offer to allow you to lead a full, productive life for a longer period of time and, indeed, to *save* your life. Consider that since the 1987 introduction of statin drugs, potent agents that lower blood cholesterol, people are living who absolutely would be dead otherwise. According to a large analysis, statins reduce heart disease risk by up to 60 percent and stroke risk by up to 17 percent.

And drugs to improve people's heart disease profile are getting better all the time. The pharmacologic gamut for heart-saving medications, in fact, is something of a moving target, with recommended drugs—and their dosages—changing as researchers continue to learn how to keep the cardiovascular system protected. For that reason, the list of drugs that follows should be thought of as a general guide (and by no means a complete one) to the current drug arsenal. Your doctor may very well tell you to take something not mentioned here, or she or he may adjust your dosage depending on such factors as what other drugs you are taking. It's okay to ask your doctor to explain her or his decision if it conflicts with what you read here or elsewhere, but in the end follow your doctor's directions. Your physician has all the particulars on you and your body, which allows for the best tailoring of drugs and drug prescriptions.

DRUGS THAT LOWER LDL-CHOLESTEROL

Medications for lowering cholesterol have undergone an amazing metamorphosis over the last twenty years, and even the last ten. To say that the arsenal of cholesterol lowerers today wasn't available when your mother was your age is a vast understatement. Sometimes two drugs with different modes of action are prescribed simultaneously for maximum effect.

Statins

With statins having changed the face of heart disease treatment, and heart disease being the biggest killer of American women as well as men, it should come as no surprise that statins are now the largest selling class of prescription medications in the United States, ahead of antidepressants, anti-heartburn agents, even pills for high blood pressure.

There are six statin drugs altogether, with more on the way. Here are their names, with the dates they began appearing on the market:

- lovastatin (Mevacor) 1987
- simastatin (Zocor) 1991
- fluvastatin (Lescol) 1993
- atorvastatin (Lipitor) 1996
- pravastatin (Pravachol) 2001
- rosuvastatin (Crestor) 2003

MODE OF ACTION: All statins work in a similar way. They inhibit cells in the liver and elsewhere from making cholesterol. That forces these cells to pull cholesterol out of the bloodstream, reducing circulating levels.

EFFICACY: People who take statins typically undergo a 20 to 60 percent reduction in LDL-cholesterol. Statins also (modestly) reduce elevated triglycerides and (modestly) increase HDL-cholesterol.

PRESCRIPTION DIRECTIONS: Some people are told to take statins with the evening meal or at bedtime. The body tends to produce more cholesterol at night than during the day. After four to eight weeks, blood cholesterol is reevaluated and the prescription adjusted, if necessary.

SIDE EFFECTS: In general, statins are very well tolerated, with a low rate of side effects. Occasionally reported are stomach upset, gas, constipation, and abdominal cramps. Fortunately, these gastrointestinal symptoms often abate with time.

More rare side effects include abnormal elevations in blood liver enzymes and muscle aches and pains. Most of the time, the rise in blood liver enzymes doesn't have any practical significance. It's reversible; the enzyme levels drop either with a lower dose or by switching to another statin.

The muscle aches and pains occur in 4 to 5 percent of people who go on statins. Sometimes they get better on their own, but they can also get worse. The effects on muscle are particularly an issue for older women.

Your doctor can sometimes correct a side-effect problem by lowering the dose or switching you to another statin. In extremely rare cases, a different class of cholesterol-lowering drug may be called for.

Resins, Also Known as Bile Acid Sequestrants

Resins were developed long before statins became available and are sometimes added to the treatment regimen if statins alone aren't doing the trick. But they don't tend to be used much anymore. They can be poorly tolerated—they have an unpleasant mouth feel and may cause constipation and bloating. For these reasons, compliance is low. There are three resin drugs:

- cholestyramine (Questan, Prevalite, Lo-Cholest)
- colestipol (Colestid)
- colesevelam (WelChol)

MODE OF ACTION: Resins do their work in the lower part of the intestine. Specifically, they bind bile acids to them, forcing them to be excreted in the stools. Why is that important? Bile acids (which are essential for dietary fat diges-

The Cause of High Cholesterol Isn't Always What You Think It Is

High cholesterol doesn't always stem from the usual culprits. In some heart disease clinics, about 5 to 10 percent of patients who have been referred by their primary care physicians actually have an underactive thyroid, which is not an uncommon cause of high cholesterol in itself. Usually, they're elderly, and often, they're women.

To lower their cholesterol, their general practitioner or internist has prescribed a statin (after suggesting changes in diet and physical activity), but it doesn't work (and may also cause statins' telltale side effects) because the problem has an unrelated cause. So the doctor sends these patients to a heart specialist to get to the bottom of what seems like an intractable problem.

A savvy doctor, however, will check a woman's thyroid before referring her to a cardiologist—particularly if she brings up that she has been feeling fatigued lately, cannot tolerate cold as well as usual, and perhaps has been constipated. These are all possible signs of a thyroid problem. If an underactive thyroid is indeed diagnosed (which is often the case), the patient is given thyroid hormone and voilà, blood cholesterol drops into the healthy range. The woman also feels a lot better all of a sudden—less fatigued, less cold, and less constipated.

tion and absorption) are made from cholesterol in the liver. Excrete them, and you force your liver to take up more cholesterol from the bloodstream in order to replace the bile acids that have been lost.

EFFICACY: Resins tend to lower LDL-cholesterol by 10 to 20 percent.

PRESCRIPTION DIRECTIONS: Resins come in powder or tablet form. They must be mixed with water or fruit juice and taken once or twice a day, with meals. Taking them with adequate fluids is important to avoid constipation, as is taking them with food to minimize side effects.

SIDE EFFECTS: Primarily gastrointestinal in nature, side effects include constipation, bloating, nausea, gas, and worsening of hemorrhoids.

Nicotinic Acid (Niacin)

Nicotinic acid, or niacin, is actually one of the B vitamins. But whereas the
amount for general dietary adequacy for women is 14 milligrams per day, it
takes thousands of milligrams (2 to 3 grams) for niacin to lower cholesterol.

Because nicotinic acid is a nutrient, it's available over the counter as a
dietary supplement. However, for the purpose of reducing elevated cholesterol, it should be taken *only* under the direction of a physician. We cannot
stress this enough. Side effects can be significant and must be carefully
monitored by a doctor.

There are two types of nicotinic acid (not to be confused with nicotin-
amide, which is also a form of niacin but cannot lower blood cholesterol):

- immediate release
- timed/extended release

MODE OF ACTION: Nicotinic acid decreases production of particles in the liver
that are necessary for carrying cholesterol and fat in the bloodstream.

EFFICACY: This drug lowers LDL-cholesterol by 10 to 20 percent. It also lowers
triglycerides—by 20 to 50 percent. And it raises the HDL-cholesterol con-
centration by 15 to 35 percent.

PRESCRIPTION DIRECTIONS: People are usually started on the immediate-release
form. To minimize side effects, doses often begin on the relatively low side
and are gradually increased to anywhere from 1.5 to 3 grams a day. If timed-
or extended-release forms are used, the dose usually tops out at 1.5 to 2.0
grams daily.

SIDE EFFECTS: There are several potential side effects. One is flushing, or hot
flashes—a result of blood vessels suddenly opening up. Some patients develop
a tolerance for the hot flashes. Others can minimize the flushing by taking

the drug with meals or aspirin (under the guidance of a physician). Timed/extended-release forms result in less flushing in some but not all people.

There can also be an increased effect of certain blood pressure medications. In some cases, nicotinic acid and blood pressure medication taken together can make blood pressure fall too low. The use of such medications must be coordinated by your physician.

Other possibilities include GI upset and an increase in liver enzymes that could signify liver dysfunction, high blood sugar (which is why it's not generally recommended for people with diabetes), and gout, which is a form of arthritis.

Ezetimibe (Zetia)

Ezetimibe, a relatively new drug, is most commonly used as an adjunct to statins when statin treatment alone is not enough to bring cholesterol levels into the desired range.

MODE OF ACTION: Whereas statins inhibit cholesterol production, ezetimibe decreases cholesterol *absorption* from the small intestine.

EFFICACY: This drug decreases LDL-cholesterol an average of 12 percent over and above what statins alone will do.

PRESCRIPTION DIRECTIONS: Ezetimibe comes in tablet form and should be taken once a day with meals or at the same time you take a statin.

SIDE EFFECTS: Adverse effects are primarily gastrointestinal and include constipation, bloating, nausea, and gas.

Plant Sterols

Naturally occurring compounds isolated from tree bark, soybeans, or other sources, plant sterols are added to certain foods—margarine, orange juice, and salad dressing, for example. They also come in softgel capsules. They are used to lower cholesterol to some degree in Finland but haven't really caught on in the United States. In this country, people seem to be hesitant about consuming foods manufactured with the express purpose of having a pharmacologic effect.

MODE OF ACTION: Plant sterols are thought to inhibit cholesterol absorption.

EFFICACY: They lower LDL-cholesterol by 10 to15 percent.

PRESCRIPTION DIRECTIONS: The average amount recommended is 1.6 to 2.0 grams a day. Levels vary among products—you may need four servings of margarine, for instance, or two cups of orange juice—so if you and your doctor decide you should go the plant sterol route, you'll need to follow the directions on the label of the food(s) you're going to use.

Note: We are not particularly enamored of the idea of putting drugs into foods, if for no other reason than once you add a food to the diet to lower cholesterol, you have to subtract calories somewhere else, so it is somewhat complicated. Also, because different foods contain different amounts of plant sterols, standardized dosing becomes difficult, if not impossible. That said, plant sterols are certainly a legitimate way to go; the National Heart, Lung, and Blood Institute has endorsed their use. If you're going to try them, we suggest you discuss with your doctor the advisability of using the softgel capsules.

SIDE EFFECTS: Generally well tolerated, plant sterols have been reported in rare cases to cause mild indigestion.

DRUGS THAT AFFECT OTHER LIPIDS

LDL-cholesterol is not the only blood lipid treated with drugs. There are also medications to raise HDL-cholesterol as well as lower triglycerides.

Fibrates

Fibrates lower elevated triglycerides. They may also raise HDL-cholesterol. (The two tend to go hand in hand.) The fibrates available are:

- genfibrozil (Lopid)
- clofibrate (Atromid-S)
- fenofibrate (Tricor)

MODE OF ACTION: Fibrates operate by increasing the rate at which triglycerides are removed from VLDL, which stands for very low-density lipoprotein.

EFFICACY: The reduction in triglyceride levels ranges from 20 to 50 percent. Elevations in HDL-cholesterol range from 10 to 15 percent.

PRESCRIPTION DIRECTIONS: Fibrates are usually given in two daily doses, thirty minutes before the morning and evening meals.

SIDE EFFECTS: These drugs are well tolerated by most patients. The most common side effect, as with many of the others, is gastrointestinal discomfort. But fibrates can also elevate the risk of developing gallstones. And they may increase the potency of anticoagulants, sometimes referred to as blood thinners, making monitoring by a physician essential.

Fish Oil Capsules

As we discussed in chapter 4, fish oil contains EPA and DHA, omega-3 fatty acids that help lower high triglycerides, make blood less "sticky" by decreasing platelet aggregation, and most important, decrease the risk of sudden cardiac death. For these reasons, as we discussed in chapter 5, everyone should be aiming for at least two fish meals a week. But some physicians advise people who have had a heart attack to take fish oil *capsules,* which have higher doses of fish oil than fish itself.

MODE OF ACTION: All the various ways in which fish oil decreases heart disease risk are not known, but researchers are aware that fish oil capsules decrease the incidence of arrhythmias and blood clotting.

EFFICACY: Three to four grams or so of fish oil a day (more than you could get in four or five fish meals) decrease triglycerides 25 to 30 percent. About 1 gram a day has been shown to decrease future heart attack risk in people who have already had a heart attack. Doctors decide how much to prescribe based on a patient's individual history.

PRESCRIPTION DIRECTIONS: While fish oil capsules are available over the counter, they should be taken only under a doctor's supervision. One reason is that while they lower triglycerides, they can also *increase* LDL-cholesterol up to 10 percent, so anyone who takes them has to be monitored.

SIDE EFFECTS: Adverse effects, which occur at levels greater than 1 gram a day, are primarily gastrointestinal in nature and include constipation, bloating, nausea, fishy belches, and gas. Excess amounts can make you prone to bleeding in the case of an accident or emergency surgery.

Does a Baby Aspirin a Day Keep the Doctor Away?

A lot of men are told by their doctors to take baby, or low-dose, aspirin regularly in order to prevent heart disease. Should women? It depends on your heart disease risk, says the American Heart Association. Given the lack of definitive evidence in women, it also depends on your physician's assessment of your particular situation. You should not buy it over the counter without her or his recommendation. Aspirin can cause gastrointestinal bleeding, and the risk of that has to be weighed against the benefit to your heart.

ASPIRIN THERAPY FOR WOMEN

at high risk: 75–162 milligrams a day* (1 to 2 baby aspirin)
at intermediate risk: 75–162 milligrams a day*
at low risk: not recommended

While the dose is the same for high and intermediate risk, a physician's decision to prescribe aspirin will depend on a woman's individual risk for side effects.

DRUGS THAT LOWER BLOOD PRESSURE

In more than two out of three people with hypertension, the condition cannot be controlled with one drug alone. Note that there are far more antihypertensive medications than drugs for cholesterol. In addition, they are frequently prescribed and sold in combination. We provide here information on general classes.

Diuretics

Diuretics, referred to by some people as "water pills," are usually the first drug of choice for people who cannot control their blood pressure through diet and exercise alone. The three major types of diuretics are thiazides, loop diuretics, and potassium-sparing diuretics.

1. Thiazides (also known as potassium-depleting diuretics)

Examples:

- chlorothiazide (Diuril)
- hydrochlorothiazide (Microzide, HydroDIURIL)
- polythiazide (Renese)
- indapamide (Lozol)
- metolazone (Mykrox)
- metolazone (Zaroxolyn)

2. Loop diuretics (also known as potassium-depleting diuretics). These are more potent than thiazide diuretics. In addition to lowering blood pressure, they are the most effective in reducing the amount of fluid volume in the body, which is good for people with congestive heart failure.

Examples:

- bumetanide (Bumex)
- furosemide (Lasix)
- torsemide (Demadex)

3. Potassium-sparing diuretics

Examples:

- amiloride (Midamor)
- triameterene (Demadex)

MODE OF ACTION: Diuretics cause the body to rid itself of excess fluids (and sodium) through urination. When there is less fluid volume in the vascular system, there is less pressure on artery walls as blood is pumped through all the blood vessels. That is, the pressure of blood in the arteries is reduced.

EFFICACY: Varies from drug to drug and patient to patient.

PRESCRIPTION DIRECTIONS: Sometimes, the recommendation for those taking potassium-depleting diuretics is to eat potassium-rich foods (see page 67 for examples). In other instances the doctor may prescribe supplemental potassium. If you miss a dose of a diuretic, wait until the next time. Do not take the dose late or double up. Diuretics should be stored at room temperature, away from moisture, light, and excess heat.

SIDE EFFECTS: Potassium-sparing diuretics can cause weakness, leg cramps, or fatigue if body potassium runs too low. But generally diuretics tend to be well tolerated (although there have been some reports of sexual dysfunction and urinary incontinence).

Angiotensin-Converting Enzyme (ACE Inhibitors)

ACE inhibitors not only can lower blood pressure but also are used to treat heart failure. Some common ACE inhibitors include:

- benazepril (Lotensin)
- captopril (Capoten)
- enalapril (Vasotec)
- fosinopril (Monopril)
- lisinopril (Prinivil, Zestril)
- moexipril (Univasc)

- perindopril (Aceon)
- quinapril (Accupril)
- ramipril (Altace)
- trandolapril (Mavik)

MODE OF ACTION: ACE inhibitors prevent the formation of a hormone called *angiotensin II,* which causes blood vessels to narrow. By "relaxing" the blood vessels, it actually allows them to expand as blood is forced out of the heart, thereby decreasing resistance to blood flowing through them. That, in turn, lowers the pressure of the blood on the artery walls. Of course, that also makes the heart's pumping work easier and more efficient. It doesn't have to pump as hard to push blood through all the arteries.

EFFICACY: Varies from drug to drug and patient to patient.

PRESCRIPTION DIRECTIONS: If you miss a dose, wait until the next time. Do not take the dose late or double up. Store at room temperature, away from moisture, light, and excess heat.

SIDE EFFECTS: Potential adverse effects, which are rare, include cough, skin rash, loss of taste, and compromised renal function. ACE inhibitors should be avoided by pregnant women.

Angiotensin II Receptor Antagonists

Angiotensin II receptor antagonists have been shown to produce blood pressure–lowering effects similar to those produced by ACE inhibitors. Current angiotensin II receptor antagonists include:

- candesartan (Atacand)
- eprosartan (Teveten)
- irbesartan (Avapro)
- losartan (Cozaar)
- oimesartan (Benicar)
- telmisartan (Micardis)
- valsartan (Diovan)

MODE OF ACTION: Whereas ACE inhibitors lower levels of angiotensin II, angiotensin II receptor antagonists prevent the blood vessel–constricting hormone from acting on cells that line the surface of blood vessels. They can be thought to "shield" blood vessels from angiotensin II.

EFFICACY: Varies from drug to drug and patient to patient.

PRESCRIPTION DIRECTIONS: If you miss a dose, wait until next time. Do not take the dose late or double up. Store at room temperature, away from moisture, light, and excess heat.

SIDE EFFECTS: Some people occasionally experience dizziness. Angiotensin II receptor antagonists should be avoided by pregnant women.

Beta-Blockers

In addition to being used to lower blood pressure, beta-blockers are sometimes prescribed to treat cardiac arrhythmias and angina and can also be useful for patients with congestive heart failure. Current beta-blockers include:

- acebutolol (Sectral)
- atenolol (Tenormin)
- betaxolol (Kerlone)
- bisoprolol (Zebeta)
- metoprolol (Lopressor)
- nadolol (Corgard)
- propranolol (Inderal)
- propranolol long-acting (Inderal-LA)
- timolol (Blocadren)

MODE OF ACTION: Beta-blockers decrease heart rate. That means that both the intervals between each pump of blood last a little longer and the heart pumps a little less intensely, cutting down on how often—and how much—pressure is exerted on the arteries as blood rushes through them.

EFFICACY: Varies from drug to drug and patient to patient.

PRESCRIPTION DIRECTIONS: If you miss a dose, wait until next time. Do not take two doses close together or double up. Store at room temperature, away from moisture, light, and excess heat.

SIDE EFFECTS: Dizziness, fatigue, insomnia, cold hands and feet, and depression have been reported, but these medications are usually well tolerated.

Calcium Channel Blockers

In addition to controlling high blood pressure, calcium channel blockers are used to treat angina and some arrhythmias. Current channel blockers on the market include:

- amlodipine (Norvasc)
- diltiazem extended release (Cardizen CD, Tiazac)
- felodipine (Plendil)
- isradipine (Dynacirc CR)
- nicardipine sustained release (Cardene SR)
- nifedipine long acting (Adalat CC, Procardia XL)
- nisoldipine (Sular)
- verapamil immediate release (Calan, Isoptin, Verelan)
- verapamil long acting (Calan SR, Isoptin SR)
- verapamil (Coer, Covera HS, Verelan PM)

MODE OF ACTION: Also known as calcium antagonists, calcium channel blockers interrupt the movement of the mineral calcium into cardiovascular cells. That causes the blood vessels to relax, which makes for less resistance; hence, there is less pressure on the artery walls as blood rushes through.

EFFICACY: Varies from drug to drug and patient to patient.

PRESCRIPTION DIRECTIONS: Take as directed. If you skip a dose, wait until next time. Do not take two doses close together or double up. Store at room temperature, away from moisture, light, and excess heat.

SIDE EFFECTS: They differ widely among drugs. Constipation, swollen ankles, headache, and dizziness are some of the more common ones.

BE SMART: LISTEN TO YOUR DOCTOR

As you can see, the arsenal of drugs available to treat cholesterol levels, other lipids, and blood pressure is enormous—and keeps getting bigger and more effective all the time. Every year, new medications reach the market.

The unfortunate truth is that not enough women are *taking* them. For example, three out of four women with high blood pressure are aware of it, but fewer than one in three are taking the necessary steps to control it. If your doctor determines that a prescription is necessary, take the drug faithfully to live as long and as healthy as possible. Comments Anne, who got her high blood pressure under control with medication, "I have a twenty-one-year-old, a seventeen-year-old, and an eleven-year-old. I fully intend to be in their lives for quite a while."

CHAPTER 10

Angioplasty, Bypass, Cardiac Catheterization: The ABCs of Medical Procedures

◆

I woke up in the middle of the night, sweating. I couldn't breathe. I called 911. When I got to the hospital, the doctor said I had had a heart attack. They did an angioplasty right then and there and put three stents in three different places to open my arteries. I had heard the term "angioplasty," but I never knew what it was. I was awake during the procedure—and scared. If I had known before about all of this, I would have had less anxiety.

—PEARL

There are times when, no matter what you do for your heart lifestyle-wise, you end up having to go through a heart-related procedure. Sometimes it's surgery; more often, it's simply a diagnostic test. Either way, it can be very scary. Tubes, anesthesia, complicated machinery and other unfamiliar medical devices, and, in this day and age, staff that may not have enough time to really explain what is happening and answer all your questions—all of that can produce a lot of anxiety on top of the anxiety a woman is already feeling if a doctor says she needs some kind of invasive test or operation.

But just knowing what it is you're being put through, for exactly what heart-saving reason, can greatly decrease the fear and anxiety about undergoing a new procedure.

What follows are some of the most common procedures—both diagnostic procedures and treatment procedures—related to the heart, including what they entail and how they help. (Similar procedures are used to predict stroke risk.) Should you end up needing one of them, you can consult this book ahead of time. Knowledge isn't just power. It's also reassurance.

Please note that procedures differ to some degree from hospital to hospital and also are being updated all the time, so the way things go may not always be exactly the way they are described here. But the explanations will serve as a reasonable heads up; you will not feel in the dark should one of these tests or operations be recommended.

DIAGNOSTIC PROCEDURES FOR CORONARY ARTERY DISEASE

Many of the diagnostic procedures listed below allow a doctor to "see" the heart or arteries—or the blood flowing through them—without actually opening you up. That is, what previously would have needed to be done with an operation can now be done with less invasive approaches.

Prior to the start of many of these procedures, risks for complications (which are very rare) will be explained. (Some people have reactions to the dyes used to see an artery during an imaging technique, for instance.) You may also be asked to sign a witnessed consent form.

Cardiac Catheterization/Coronary Angiography

If you're feeling chest pain upon even light exertion such as walking up the stairs, your doctor may send you for this procedure. It provides information on blood pressure within the heart; how much oxygen is in the blood flowing through the heart and coronary arteries; and the heart's pumping ability. Cardiac catheterization is often performed in tandem with coronary angioplasty (see page 195).

HOW IT WORKS: First, an intravenous line is inserted into a blood vessel through either the groin or an arm. Then, under the guidance of X-rays, a catheter, or thin tube, is inserted right through the intravenous line to the location in the heart or blood vessel that's of interest (that's the catheterization part). Next, a dye is inserted into the catheter (the angiography part). Because it's of a color-contrast material, the dye is visible with X-rays and thereby gives an indication of whether, or to what degree, your blood is flowing, or more important, *where* blood flow is impeded or partially blocked. For instance, it can show how much of an artery's diameter is closed off due to plaque or other blockages.

BEFORE THE PROCEDURE: Usually, you will be told to restrict food and fluid for a period of time before the test.

About thirty minutes prior to the catheterization, you may be given a mild sedative. You'll also be told to lie flat on your back, and the area where the catheter will be inserted will be cleansed. A local anesthetic will be used to numb the site where the IV will be inserted.

DURING THE PROCEDURE: You will be awake throughout the procedure. Because blood vessels do not have nerve endings, it is unlikely that you will feel the catheter while the angiography is being performed. You may simply feel some pressure at the site where the catheter is inserted and, since the procedure can last from one to several hours, you may feel some discomfort from having to remain in one position for that length of time.

AFTER THE PROCEDURE: When the catheter is removed, firm pressure will be applied at the site of insertion to prevent bleeding. If the catheter was inserted in the groin, you will likely be asked to remain lying on your back for a few hours after the procedure to avoid bleeding.

Electrocardiogram (ECG, EKG)

An electrocardiogram measures the electrical activity of the heart, which allows for an assessment of the heart rate and the regularity of heartbeats. It can also assess the size of the heart chambers, the presence of any damage to the heart muscle, and the effects of drugs or devices used to regulate the heart.

HOW IT WORKS The doctor or doctor's assistant will affix electrodes—little disks—to your arms, legs, and chest while you are in the reclining position. The number of electrodes varies, ranging from as few as three to five to as many as twelve to fifteen. The electrodes measure the heart's electrical activity, which allows for an assessment of electric pulsations associated with the heart's squeezing, or pumping, function. The measurements are indicated with a series of blips on a long line inked onto a piece of paper or imaged on a computer screen. Different patterns or intervals in those blips indicate how long electrical waves take to pass from one part of the heart to the other. Read by trained personnel, the patterns provide information on how your heart is functioning.

BEFORE THE PROCEDURE: There are no restrictions on consumption of food or medications prior to this procedure. Simply, the areas where the electrodes will be placed will be cleansed.

DURING THE PROCEDURE: You may feel a little cold at the sites where the disks are attached. You will not feel anything else since the EKG machine to which the electrodes are attached is only measuring electrical impulses normally going through your heart. The whole procedure takes about five minutes.

AFTER THE PROCEDURE: In rare circumstances, a rash or irritation may develop at the sites where the disks were attached.

Echocardiogram (Transthoracic Echocardiogram; Doppler Ultrasound of the Heart)

An echocardiogram is an ultrasound of the heart, meaning that sound waves are used to create a two-dimensional picture of the heart muscle as it pumps and squeezes. (Think of how an ultrasound allows a developing fetus to be seen as it moves about in the uterus.) The picture, which is much more detailed than what an X-ray could provide, allows a physician (usually a cardiologist) to view the valves, walls, and chambers of the heart in a noninvasive manner. It also allows assessment of movement to evaluate pumping capacity or flow characteristics. Specifically, echocardiograms allow doctors to assess heart murmurs, check the pumping strength and efficiency of the heart, and check up on patients who have had a heart attack.

HOW IT WORKS: An instrument called a transducer is placed on various spots on the chest and directed toward the heart. The transducer sends out high-frequency sound waves and then picks up their echoes, which will change based on the heart's structure and function. It then transmits the echoes as electrical impulses to a computerized echocardiography machine that converts them into actual pictures of the heart.

BEFORE THE PROCEDURE: No special preparation is required.

DURING THE PROCEDURE: No dyes or X-rays are involved. A gel will be spread on your chest, and the transducer will then be applied. You will feel a slight pressure from the transducer but nothing else. You may be asked to breathe in a certain way or to roll over onto your left side.

AFTER THE PROCEDURE: You should feel no different from before the procedure.

Exercise Stress Test

An exercise stress test assesses the effect of exercise on your heart. In some cases, it may be ordered by your physician when you talk to her or him about starting an exercise program. More often, it is performed to determine whether you have blockages in the arteries supplying your heart, to determine your exercise capacity, or to identify heart rate rhythm disturbances during exercise.

Often, the heart is imaged both just before and during or immediately after a stress test, which strengthens diagnostic accuracy. This is particularly important for women, who tend to have higher episodes of false positives on standard stress tests than men. Imaging is generally done with either echocardiography or what is known as nuclear scanning. Sometimes with echocardiography but always with nuclear scanning, an IV is inserted in the arm before exercise begins and special substances infused that facilitate imaging of the blood supplying the heart as well as the heart's pumping action.

HOW IT WORKS: Essentially, an electrocardiogram is performed while you walk (or run) on a treadmill or pedal on a stationary bicycle. These conditions are intended to simulate a situation in which your heart needs to respond to the demand for extra oxygen.

BEFORE THE PROCEDURE: Your heath care provider will give you instructions, which frequently involve not eating or drinking for about three hours before the test. Wear comfortable, loose-fitting clothing and appropriate shoes. Electrodes will be attached to your chest, arms, and legs. A blood pressure cuff will be placed around one arm.

DURING THE PROCEDURE: You will be asked to walk, run, or pedal, usually until you reach a target heart rate or you can't continue because you are too tired. Your heart rate and blood pressure will be monitored throughout the procedure. Sometimes, if you experience chest pain or your blood pressure increases precipitously during the test, you will be told to stop.

AFTER THE PROCEDURE: Heart rate and blood pressure are usually monitored for ten to fifteen minutes after you complete the exercise. You will likely feel the blood pressure cuff inflate and deflate at regular intervals.

Besides possibly feeling a little tired, you should not feel any different after you complete a stress test. In rare circumstances, a rash or irritation may develop at the sites where the disks were attached.

Myocardial Biopsy

A myocardial biopsy is often performed if cardiomyopathy (inflammation of the heart muscle) or cardiac amyloidosis (deposition of abnormal proteins in the heart muscle) is suspected. It's also conducted after a heart transplant to detect potential rejection of the new heart tissue.

HOW IT WORKS: Small pieces of heart muscle (usually three to five) are removed for examination.

BEFORE THE PROCEDURE: Several days before the test, you will likely be told to stop taking aspirin or other medications that affect bleeding time. You will be asked to restrict food and fluid intake for six to eight hours before the procedure. A mild sedative will be given to you about thirty minutes before the biopsy takes place. You will be asked to lie flat on your back. Local anesthesia will be applied at the spot where a catheter will be inserted.

DURING THE PROCEDURE: As with a cardiac catheterization, you will be awake throughout. If cardiac tissue is needed from the right ventricle, a catheter is inserted through a vein (usually the jugular vein in the neck, sometimes with X-rays to guide the catheter). If it's needed from the left ventricle, it's inserted through an artery. Either way, a jaw-like apparatus on the tip of the catheter is used to snip off small pieces of heart muscle tissue.

AFTER THE PROCEDURE: You will have some pressure applied to the site where the catheter was inserted in order to prevent bleeding.

TREATMENT PROCEDURES

All of these procedures require admittance to the hospital, either as a day-patient or as an in-patient. Leave all your jewelry (including rings, if possible) and other valuables at home. You will be asked to sign a witnessed consent form to acknowledge your understanding that there are rare cases of complications.

Angioplasty (Balloon Angioplasty)

Angioplasty is performed to widen a blood vessel that has been narrowed, or blocked, by atherosclerotic plaque. The blockage is often discovered during a coronary angiography, and the angioplasty (often in tandem with a cardiac catheterization) is performed right then, with the aim of increasing blood flow to the compromised area. The end result is relief from chest pain and improved exercise capacity.

HOW IT WORKS: A catheter with an inflatable balloon at the tip is inserted into the narrowed artery. It is then positioned right in or near the atherosclerotic blockage and inflated, which widens the blood vessel and restores adequate blood flow.

BEFORE THE PROCEDURE: Usually, you will be told to restrict food and fluid for a period of time before the test. About thirty minutes prior to the catheterization, you may be given a mild sedative. You'll also be told to lie flat on your back, and the area where the catheter will be inserted will be cleansed. A local anesthetic will be given to numb the site, and the catheter will then be inserted (usually near the groin but sometimes in the arm or even the neck).

DURING THE PROCEDURE: An antiplatelet drug will be administered to minimize the risk of forming a blood clot. As the blocked blood vessel is opened and blood starts flowing smoothly once again, a *stent,* which is nothing more than a wire-mesh tube, is sometimes placed at the site as a kind of scaffolding to ensure that the area remains open. It remains in place permanently.

AFTER THE PROCEDURE: Pressure will be applied to the site where the catheter was inserted to avoid bleeding. You will have to lie still for several hours to allow the blood vessels at the point of entry to seal completely. The area may remain sore for up to one week, although you will usually leave the hospital the next day or the day after. When you are discharged, you will be given guidelines on what you may and may not do once you return home.

Angioplasty Variations

Percutaneous Transmyocardial Coronary Angioplasty (Transmyocardial Revascularization)

This procedure is usually performed to relieve severe angina or chest pain in very ill patients who aren't candidates for bypass surgery or traditional angioplasty. A surgeon makes an incision in the breast, exposing the heart. With a laser, she or he then drills several small holes into the heart's pumping chamber. How this procedure helps is unclear. It may be that the laser stimulates the growth of new blood vessels by causing bleeding. Another theory is that the laser destroys nerve fibers to the heart, which could reduce pain.

Laser Angioplasty

Approved by the Food and Drug Administration in 1992 and available at some of the larger medical centers, laser angioplasty is still in the developmental stage. Once in place at or near the blockage, the laser emits pulsating beams of light that vaporize the plaque.

Bypass Surgery

If blockage in an artery is severe or if blockages are too widespread for angioplasty and stenting, coronary artery bypass surgery will likely be necessary. Women who undergo bypass surgery sometimes have angina prior to the operation; that is what brings them in to see their physician. They may have a feeling of heaviness, tightness, pain, pressure, squeezing, or any of the most general symptoms of a heart attack. However, symptoms in women are often subtle, and only diagnostic testing leads to the discovery of disease advanced enough to require the surgery.

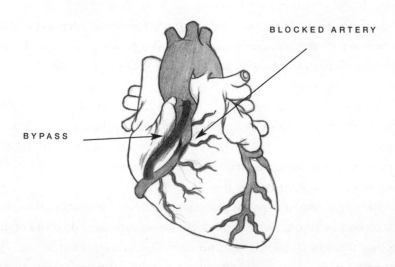

Bypass surgery: A vein from a breast or leg is grafted onto a coronary artery above and below the blockage.

HOW IT WORKS: Also known as a coronary artery bypass graft, or CABG ("cabbage"), bypass surgery is just that. It uses a blood vessel from the leg or chest to bypass (go around) a coronary artery that is blocked by atherosclerotic plaque. That allows the heart muscle to be nourished with blood it was otherwise deprived of.

BEFORE THE PROCEDURE: Because you will be under general anesthesia, you will be instructed not to eat or drink for eight to twelve hours before the surgery.

DURING THE PROCEDURE: The traditional approach during bypass has been for the patient to be connected to a heart-lung machine that does the work of those two organs for the duration of the operation; the heart's beating is temporarily stopped while blood flows through the machine instead. But that creates potential complications in the way of declines in memory and mental clarity, lung and kidney complications, and an increased risk for stroke. A newer approach, called *off-pump coronary artery bypass* or simply *minimally invasive heart surgery* (see below), allows the heart to keep pumping during the surgery and also avoids opening the chest.

AFTER THE PROCEDURE: Heart rate and blood pressure will be monitored continuously for twelve to twenty-four hours. A urinary catheter and IV will remain in place until you're stable. An endotracheal tube will also stay in place until you are awake and can breathe comfortably on your own.

The incision in the chest and graft sites will be uncomfortable for forty-eight to seventy-two hours. You will be provided painkillers as needed.

You may spend three to five days in the hospital, with the first couple of hours in intensive care. You may have some "fuzzy thinking" during that time.

A cardiac rehabilitation program should begin when your doctor, in consultation with you, feels it's appropriate—sometimes while you're in the hospital but often after you return home.

When you do get back home, you may have loss of appetite, constipation, swelling at areas of incision, fatigue, mood swings, and difficulty sleeping. These side effects, which don't affect everybody, can last four to six weeks. Usually, you can resume sexual activity four weeks after the surgery and return to work in four to six weeks. The full benefits of the operation can take as long as three to six months to be realized, although sometimes sooner. Many people report feeling much better than they have in years.

Bypass Variation: Minimally Invasive Heart Surgery

With this type of bypass, the heart continues beating during the operation. This allows the procedure to be performed without a heart-lung machine, making the operation safer than traditional bypass surgery. The patient tends to require fewer blood transfusions, has a decreased risk of stroke, a shorter postoperative hospital stay, and a shorter recovery period. There are two main types:

Minimally Invasive Direct Coronary Bypass
This is for blockages in a coronary artery located in the front of the heart. A small incision (2 to 4 inches) is made in the left chest before the procedure is performed.

Off-Pump Coronary Artery Bypass
A vertical incision the size of the incision for traditional bypass surgery is made in the chest, and the breastbone is split to allow access to the entire heart. A stabilizing device is put over the section of the beating heart to restrict movement where the blockage will be bypassed.

Heart Valve Surgery

As you'll recall from chapter 2, heart valves keep blood flowing in the right direction through the heart's chambers. But they need to be repaired or replaced if they leak blood backward (*regurgitation*) or become too narrow to let sufficient blood pass (*stenosis*). Defective valves that are not dealt with may cause congestive heart failure. Heart valve problems can originate in a number of ways: via infections, such as rheumatic fever; birth defects; calcification (hardening of the actual valve); or from certain medications (the weight-loss drug combination Fen-Phen, for example).

Save Someone *Else's* Life

Nearly everyone is familiar with the paddles and crash cart associated with TV dramas. When the crash cart is called for, an electric shock is delivered to a patient's heart during cardiac arrest or if the heart is experiencing arrhythmia. This can reestablish normal contractions (rhythms) in the heart, allowing the patient to survive a life-and-death situation.

The medical term for the procedure is *defibrillation,* and now people without formal medical training can be taught to use automated external defibrillators (AEDs), standard equipment today in airports, convention centers, and other facilities where large numbers of people congregate. Local chapters of both the Red Cross and the American Heart Association teach people how to safely and effectively use AEDs.

In addition, they teach standard cardiopulmonary resuscitation (CPR). CPR has been the mainstay of keeping alive someone who has stopped breathing or whose heart has stopped pumping while you await professional help.

While saving your own life through eating better and getting more physical activity, you might just want to learn how to save someone else's in an emergency.

HOW IT WORKS: Repair or replacement of a faulty valve usually requires open-heart surgery. Repair entails restoring the functioning of the existing valve. A surgeon will try to repair your own valve whenever possible. Replacement uses either a *biologic* valve—one obtained from a human cadaver or modified from a pig or cow valve—or an *artificial* valve made from synthetic materials.

BEFORE THE PROCEDURE: Because you will be under general anesthesia, you will be instructed not to eat or drink for eight to twelve hours before the surgery.

DURING THE PROCEDURE: You will be connected to a heart-lung machine that does the work of those two organs for the duration of the operation; the heart's beating is temporarily stopped while blood flows through the machine instead. The old valve is repaired, or it is removed and the new one is sewn into place.

AFTER THE PROCEDURE: You will spend two to three days in the intensive care unit so heart function can be monitored continuously, then another week or two in a regular patient room. You may notice an occasional "clicking noise" or sensation in your chest the first days after surgery if an artificial replacement valve (not human, porcine, or bovine) is used. This should occur less often with time and go away completely within the first couple of weeks. (If it gets worse, call your doctor.) Bear in mind that it may take months to feel back to yourself, depending on your health before the surgery. Also, note that you will need to take anticoagulant therapy for at least several months—and for the rest of your life if you have a replacement valve that is artificial. And you must always take antibiotics before dental or surgical procedures because of an increased risk for developing an infection of the valve (endocarditis).

Pacemaker

A small, battery-operated electronic device, a pacemaker is inserted under the skin in the chest to help the heart beat regularly and at an appropriate rate. It's commonly used when the natural pacing or conduction system of the heart no longer functions properly. A pacemaker senses when the heart rate is getting too slow or too fast and shifts the rate in the appropriate direction. It also helps the heart to beat more efficiently, adding to pumping capacity in those with weakened heart performance, such as people with congestive heart failure.

HOW IT WORKS: Wires go from a generator through a large vein to the heart, sending electrical impulses that cause the heart to beat. The generator contains the battery as well as the "information" for regulating the heartbeat and weighs only about 1 ounce. The battery lasts seven to eight years.

BEFORE THE PROCEDURE: Usually you will be told to restrict food and fluid for a period of time before the procedure.

DURING THE PROCEDURE: Inserting a pacemaker takes approximately one hour. You will be awake but given pain medication. A small incision is made in the chest, and a small pocket underneath the skin is created. Then, using guidance via X-rays, leads are positioned in the heart, from where they are connected to the generator. Finally, the pacemaker is placed in the pocket and the incision is closed.

AFTER THE PROCEDURE: People who have a pacemaker must carry an identification card—in case they ever lose consciousness. They must also notify people operating certain common devices because those devices—electronic anti-theft surveillance systems, metal detectors, MRI machines, and therapeutic radiation apparatus for treating cancer—can throw off the pacemaker's electric signals. (Home appliances carry little to no risk.)

Pacemaker Variation: Internal Defibrillator
Internal defibrillators are sometimes implanted in people who are very vulnerable to life-threatening heart rhythm disturbances. A personalized, micro-mini version of a crash cart and paddles, it jolts the heart whenever necessary.

CARDIAC REHABILITATION:
A KEY TO LONG-TERM RECOVERY

While not technically a procedure, cardiac rehabilitation is the culmination of many procedures that people go through—or the culmination of aggressive treatment they may have received in the wake of a heart attack or other serious cardiovascular problem. Simply put, it is a professionally guided program to teach women and men heart-healthy lifestyle habits that includes a prescriptive exercise program once their heart disease has been tended to medically.

It has been estimated that cardiac rehabilitation could prevent the premature deaths of hundreds of thousands of people. But here's the irony:

While the United States is the best place in the world to be if you're in the throes of a heart attack or need intricate surgery to clear a clogged artery (or bypass one that's too far gone), low-tech and low-cost cardiac rehabilitation is underutilized. Only 10 to 20 percent of those eligible actually end up participating.

Why? In large part, the medical community to date has been more devoted to aggressive treatment of an existing cardiovascular problem than to prevention of further problems down the road. Not enough people are referred.

We believe that approach needs rethinking. Cardiac rehabilitation is a golden opportunity not just to avoid a second heart attack or angioplasty but also to receive what's essentially a personalized health makeover. In cardiac rehabilitation, you meet with various health care professionals over several weeks or months who coordinate with your physician to help you quit smoking, if necessary; work out an individualized weight-loss plan, if you are overweight; and develop the right "mix" of diet, drugs, and physical activity (you are usually assigned a trainer) to help keep down blood pressure, blood cholesterol, and blood sugar. Even mental health is addressed, with classes in stress management and the like.

We strongly urge you to lobby for cardiac rehabilitation should you find yourself in the hospital for a serious cardiovascular problem or procedure. In most cases, all you need is your physician's referral.

Note that once you have a referral in hand, insurance coverage or geographic location may limit your choice of programs. If possible, try to enter a program that has been certified by the American Association of Cardiovascular and Pulmonary Rehabilitation. That means it meets standards for having appropriately trained staff—and for measuring your progress with appropriate tests.

Incidentally, Pearl, the woman quoted at the beginning of this chapter, was lucky enough to be referred to cardiac rehabilitation right after her heart attack. Because of it, she never smoked another cigarette—and learned a fair amount about exercise and diet, too.

CHAPTER 11

It's *Your* Turn!

◆

If I had known then what I know now, I would have put up much more of a ruckus than I did.

—DeLinda

One night in January, DeLinda recounts, "I woke in the middle of the night. I just didn't feel right. I was really cold up around my shoulders. I was having trouble breathing. You know when there's just something not right in your body."

DeLinda's husband started to drive her to the hospital. But she was feeling so poorly that they stopped at the local fire station. And none too soon. Her blood pressure had spiked to 225 over 110, and her pulse rate was 44—too low for someone who's not an athlete.

The fire department took DeLinda to the emergency room, where the nightmare she was going through began to take on a new dimension. "They gave me some blood pressure medication and referred me to my primary care doctor," she says. "They just kind of sloughed me off as having an anxiety attack."

The next morning, DeLinda phoned her doctor but had to leave a message. When he called back, she was on the line. The voice mail message he left was: "I do not have time to play phone tag."

Making matters worse still, various medications DeLinda's doctors had prescribed to lower her blood pressure weren't working well enough. After a number of feeling-sick, off-hour visits to the emergency room, she was finally referred to a cardiologist. The cardiologist put her on a new drug that did help, but for almost two months, DeLinda was too weak to go to work.

It was totally out of character, her daughter, Kim, says. "My mother's not one to lie around."

DeLinda then pushed herself to go back to work despite not feeling right (she's the manager of a high-end shoe store), and then one day in mid-March, she began "feeling really funny in my chest. It wasn't horrible pain. It was more of a burning sensation. I started to go to the hospital. It stopped. I went back to work. I thought, Maybe it's in my head.

"Then the owner of the company came in and said, 'You don't look good.'" He drove DeLinda to the hospital, where she was told she had bronchitis and prescribed an antibiotic. Her pain at that point was coming in waves. "One of the nurses thought I had indigestion," DeLinda recalls. "I told her I didn't. She asked me, 'Do you want to be sick?'"

At eleven o'clock that night, DeLinda sat straight up in bed and said to her husband, 'Andy, I am dying.'"

She was doubled over. Andy said he had never seen anyone in so much pain in his life.

He got her to the emergency room, where she was made to wait for an hour and a half, throwing up and moaning and crying in agony, until she was finally brought to an examining room. An EKG showed she was having a massive heart attack. She was then airlifted to a metropolitan hospital, where she stopped breathing on the table—"they called Code Blue" and "paged the chaplain," Kim says. DeLinda was brought back to life with paddles. One of her main coronary arteries was completely blocked.

She is back to work, but only half time. "She's still a lot more tired than she typically is," Kim says. "Before, she was always ready to go do something. Now she has to sit down even in the middle of getting herself dressed. There was a lot of damage done to her heart."

There is no excuse for what happened to DeLinda (who went on to cardiac rehabilitation). She knew something was wrong, her family knew, and even her medical records showed it. This was in 2004, not forty years ago or even ten years ago. Yet no one in a position to help was paying close enough attention. Now, she is paying a very high price. Indeed, at 61, she almost paid the ultimate price.

You never know what your particular circumstances are going to be, but

we believe it's possible to help keep things from getting so far out of hand—
through advocacy. To get the best out of the health care system, it's crucial
that you take an active role and advocate for yourself. DeLinda, with 20/20
hindsight, wholeheartedly agrees. "I would have gotten to the doctor sooner
in the first place," she says. "I waited too long. It was the holidays. I told
myself, 'It'll go away.'" She also feels she didn't trust her own instincts enough
to speak up when she needed to. "What women have to do is listen to their
bodies," she notes. "I was taking them at their word. I would definitely speak
to the doctors differently if this happened now. I would stay in the doctor's
office until I got answers to my questions."

A lot of women are not comfortable being vocal self-advocates. Women
are brought up to be accommodating, respectful, never questioning the status quo or rocking the boat. Women are typically conflict avoiders. But you
cannot live a respectful life without first respecting *yourself* to make sure you
get the best care possible. Indeed, if you don't treat yourself respectfully, it
can *cost* you your life.

It takes courage to advocate for yourself, especially if you're not used to it.
But *there are no boundaries to what you can do for yourself if you speak up for
your own cause.* It doesn't mean that you have to be rude, but it does mean
holding firm. You don't have to take your care or your situation at face value.
DeLinda was in no way responsible for the poor and sometimes callous
medical treatment she received, but if she had known how to work the
system better, perhaps she would have gotten the help she needed months
earlier and avoided a lot of heart muscle damage.

That's what this chapter is about: working the system through advocating
for yourself. You need to find the fortitude for that within your own mind;
with friends and family; with your doctor and other health care professionals; and, if necessary, at the hospital.

HOW YOU TALK TO YOURSELF

The most important discussion you're ever going to have about your heart
health is the one you have with yourself. For better or worse, *you* are the one
who's ultimately responsible for your own primary care. Everything else

flows from that. Of course, if you're reading this book, you've already been having that most important internal dialogue and taking the reins to your own health. By learning what you can do for yourself lifestyle-wise to protect your heart and also by learning a lot of the technical terminology related to heart health and heart disease, you have put yourself in a better position to have meaningful interactions with your health care providers—doctors, nurses, and so on.

But you also need a plan to put your knowledge into action; change doesn't come easily. Even something as simple as making sure to eat at least seven servings of vegetables and fruit a day is not a snap if you've spent decades following a different kind of eating pattern. You also need to plan regular doctor's visits; that's a crucial part of living a healthful lifestyle.

It's simple enough to make a plan. You write it down so you can check off what you've accomplished as you go along. It's how you talk to yourself about your plan—how you do or do not advocate for yourself—that can get in the way.

Psychologists talk about it in terms of triggers. There are five types of triggers: cognitive, emotional, environmental, physical, and social. They can be positive or negative, depending on whether they enhance your ability to do something for yourself or interfere.

For instance, a negative *cognitive* trigger, which is a trigger based on how you think about your predicament, would be: "I don't have time to exercise." That might seem irrefutable—after all, most women lead busy lives. But a way around it might be to actually sit down with a calendar or day planner and see where it would be possible to wedge in exercise. Perhaps it comes down to missing a certain television show a few nights a week, getting up a little earlier several times a week, getting a neighbor to watch the kids for an hour here or there, or joining a gym on your commuting route. Whatever the answer, "I don't have time to exercise" becomes a different tape playing in your head because you no longer accept it as a given and actively look for ways to work exercise into what is probably an already-packed schedule.

A negative *emotional* trigger might be guilt—which is very common in people who want to make a change but don't. The guilt ends up sucking up all the emotional energy that should be going toward the change, when it would be better for a woman to tell herself that even a small change, such as eating another vegetable every day or using the stairs for three flights, is a start. It's amazing how one small step leads to another until there's significant momentum, and the guilt is very effectively replaced with actions that, before long, turn into habits.

It's the same for *environmental, physical,* and *social* triggers. If your home environment is such that caloric treats high in saturated or *trans* fat are always around instead of fruit and low-fat yogurt, *of course* your environment is going to work against you. If, on the other hand, you feel like having cake, candy, or ice cream but the only options in the house are plain nonfat yogurt topped with berries or already-cut watermelon chunks and pineapple rings, your environment can't sabotage your efforts. (If it's not a black-and-white issue because others in the household are not as committed as you are to following a heart-healthy diet, you may have to set up "safe zones" in the cabinets or refrigerator shelves to minimize temptation. The degree to which such artificial barriers can help is amazing. They keep your priorities in the front of your mind.)

If *physically* speaking, you always feel too tired to take care of yourself by exercising, you need to remind yourself that while anticipating making changes to your exercise pattern can seem exhausting and may even feel very tiring at first, people who get some physical activity most days of the week and also eat right report feeling heightened energy after just a short time. Similarly, making the necessary dietary changes may seem like work at the beginning—you have to get used to grocery shopping and preparing food regularly—but once they become the "default" mode, they are no more time-consuming than the habits you currently have.

Finally, if your *social* triggers are holding you back—your friends would rather sit around over a mocha latte rather than take a walk—it's important not to let them stand in your way. (More on that shortly.)

It's all about finding your *inner strength*. You need to advocate for yourself when another part of you is whispering undermining messages in your ear. It's crucial, because it not only lets you live more healthfully, it also lets you speak up for yourself to others when you need to. When you are strong you'll never let the inclination to be polite stand in the way of your health.

To help you become your own best advocate, to be assertive about taking care of yourself properly, here are some questions to ask yourself. They sound simple on the surface but get to the root of taking the bull by the horns.

- When was the last time I went to the doctor for a thorough physical? (If it has been longer than two years, make an appointment now.)
- When am I going to get to the store to buy some new athletic shoes?
- When am I going to exercise this week? Which days work for me? What time of day can I fit it in? (By all means get out your calendar or date book and write it down. Don't just go through it in your head.)
- What errands can I do this week by walking instead of driving?
- What strategy can I use to ensure that I follow my "kitchen closed" policy after dinner? How will I handle it if someone else in the house has a snack after I'm done eating for the evening? With what will I replace eating while watching television?
- How can I buy the most wholesome take-out dinners on evenings that I know I won't have time to cook? How will I ensure appropriate portion control once I get those meals home? Will I put half in the refrigerator before I sit down to eat? Will I dole out a portion that's supposedly meant for one person to two or even three people in the household?
- At what time of day can I take twenty minutes to just sit and relax, read my book, or meditate?

HOW YOU TALK TO OTHERS IN YOUR CIRCLE

Once you've embraced the idea that you're going to be your own best advocate, it's important to let others know where you stand—and bring them on board, if possible. In the best of all possible worlds, your spouse or others with whom you are close are totally with you, happy to go along with changes you want to make to the meals and snacks that come out of the kitchen along with scheduling changes to accommodate your exercise regimen.

But a lot of spouses and others close to you are simply not buy-ins. You have to make decisions for yourself, even if your husband, partner, children, or friends don't want to go along. That doesn't mean you have a bad marriage or family life or even unsupportive significant others. But it probably does mean that you'll have to do things a little differently from others in your life—and not backtrack because you don't want to seem like a spoiled sport.

After all, if your loved ones have a right to their lifestyle habits without running them by you first, you have a right to yours.

By the same token, your family and friends are entitled to their latte, if they want it. You need to be clear with them that you are committed to your lifestyle changes and that they have to respect you enough to support you in your efforts, even if they don't want to join in. But you don't need to start preaching. In fact, you can even order a coffee with skim milk during the latte fests so as not to lose out on good socializing. A woman can work within *any* situation if she prepares ahead of time.

Sometimes, your new resolve may even interest some otherwise uninterested parties in making heart-healthy changes themselves. Whether or not that happens, it pays to work at actively identifying other people in your life who might be good candidates for becoming more directly involved in helping you meet your heart-health goals—or who at least will not try to hold you back from doing what you need to do because it changes the status quo. It's easier if you don't go it totally alone.

The most obvious and natural pool of people outside your home are your friends, coworkers, or other family members you count among your friends—siblings, grown children, and so on. Maybe they'll want to exercise with you, or share recipes with you, or just be willing to engage in a running dialogue with you about the strides you're making and the hurdles you have to cross.

Like-minded people can come from a broader circle, too. It's easier than you think. Maybe you'll start talking to a neighbor you frequently see on her daily walk. Or perhaps you'll find someone who walks regularly at work during lunchtime and ask if you can join her.

Sometimes you may want to *hire* players for your "support group." Maybe it's a good time to make an appointment with a psychotherapist who can help you work through some old issues that have kept you from moving ahead. Maybe paying for several sessions with a personal trainer to help you get the hang of strength training is what you need to jump-start your exercise efforts.

Whether the person or people are part of your social network or professionals you pay for their expertise, enlisting others in your cause is one of the best ways to take care of yourself and make sure you're *getting taken care of* at the same time.

Indeed, having people in your corner can enhance your actual medical care. DeLinda's daughter, Kim, for instance, remembers that her mother "started feeling extremely tired and short of breath" earlier than she herself remembers—important information for medical professionals in their assessment and treatment. She knew, too, that the problem must be her mother's heart even when others were not identifying it. "I'm no doctor," Kim says. "But you go to a reputable site on the Internet. You do a little research. You put two and two together." In other words, having someone on your team can encourage you to keep seeking treatment even when you and others around you have doubts.

Kim only wishes, in fact, that she had advocated *more* strongly for her mother—and certainly wouldn't hesitate to do so in the future. Having been there for some of the emergency room visits, she says that if she could do it over again, "I would have kept asking, 'What is causing all this pain and discomfort?' I would have pressed more. I felt this incredible sense of frustration.

"My brother's wife is a nurse. She told me, 'You're going to have to ask questions and keep asking, and push and push and push.'" Now Kim knows just how true those words of advice were.

Following are some things you might say to those in your inner circle to make sure you get what you need from them:

- *To a friend:* I am starting a walking program and can't think of someone I'd rather walk with than you. Would you consider making a commitment to walk with me for a half hour just two times a week? I don't mean a stroll; I really need to *walk.* But we can still talk and connect during that time.
- *To a husband and children:* I need you to stop making fun of my new choices. I'm not telling you that you can't snack on whatever you'd like. But I deserve the same respect. If you can't be on my side in this, at least don't try to sabotage my efforts.
- *To coworkers:* I know I've never ordered this way before when we've gone out to lunch. But I'm really trying to make an effort to eat better for heart health. Please don't give me a hard time. I need your support right now.
- *To kids:* If you see the bedroom door closed, unless it is an emergency, please wait twenty minutes. I need that uninterrupted time to unwind.

- *To family:* I would like to take a vacation this year that allows me to be more active with hiking and bicycling. But I know you guys love to loll on the beach. Let's choose a place that will meet all our wishes.
- *To a yoga instructor:* I have high cholesterol and am really stressed out. What can you tell me about your class? What are the other participants like? I'm beginning an exercise program, but are they all starting out fitter than I am? I need to push myself, but I have to be comfortable enough to be able to stick with it—and enjoy it.

HOW YOU TALK TO YOUR DOCTOR

Despite her regrets about not speaking up more for herself during her medical nightmare, there is one way DeLinda took care of herself that she is very pleased with. She switched primary care physicians after it was clear her doctor was not the one for her. Once the two of them did finally speak about her symptoms after the "phone tag" incident, DeLinda says that "he treated me like, 'Get over it.' I never went back."

It was actually her new primary care physician who referred her to a cardiologist. The medication he had prescribed was not bringing down her blood pressure adequately and he told her point-blank, "I'm not trained to deal with what's going on."

DeLinda is very glad about having made the decision to change doctors. But there's more to getting the most out of your medical team than respecting yourself enough not to accept anything less than respect from others. And there's more than asking the right questions and not backing down during a crisis. There's also advocating for yourself by talking with your doctor and asking the right questions *all along.*

Imagine if your doctor told you that you had high cholesterol and wanted to see you in six weeks to retest it—and said that if your cholesterol didn't come down, she or he was going to prescribe statin drugs. Then, imagine if you walked in after six weeks and said, "I've lost five pounds, I'm walking almost every day, and I'm eating more fruits and vegetables and fewer heavy desserts. If my cholesterol is coming down but still is not low enough, what else can I do?"

A lot will have changed in your relationship with your health care provider. One thing is that most assuredly your physician will listen to you and be much more willing to work *with* you rather than "from above." Perhaps even more important, *you'll* feel emboldened—and less flustered by the prospect of being in the doctor's office. You'll also expect more from your doctor because you will have expected more from yourself. You'll be more inclined to ask yourself, either consciously or unconsciously, "Is my doctor up to the mark?"

It's important to write down your questions before going to the doctor's office so you don't end up forgetting something that's important to you. In this day and age of managed care, doctors are under tremendous time constraints, and the better prepared you are, the better use you'll be able to make of what might be a short visit. The two of us are strong women who have no problem speaking up for ourselves when we see our doctors, but still, each of us writes down a list of questions to ask so that we get the most out of our visits. For many, it also cuts down on nervousness.

Some questions you might want to ask your health care provider:

- *What are my numbers?* Everyone should be aware of her blood lipids (cholesterol and triglycerides) and blood pressure. Even if they're in the desirable range, you want to know if they're going up. You want to be able to assess risk for yourself. By the same token, you want to know if your lifestyle measures are working and the numbers are going down—and to what degree. Ask for a copy of your reports.
- *Can I get sessions with a dietitian?* If your cholesterol, triglycerides, blood pressure, or glucose is high, and you're overweight or simply aware that you need to follow a more healthful diet but don't know how, counseling with a registered dietitian can help bring your numbers into line—often without drugs. With many health insurance companies, a referral from your doctor makes the sessions free (or free plus a small co-payment).
- *Are there diagnostic tests I should be getting to make sure we know the root of the problem?* (For instance, as we explained in chapter 9, high LDL-cholesterol is sometimes a sign of a thyroid problem rather than a cardiovascular problem, meaning a simple blood test might be in order.)

- *Should I also be seeing a cardiologist?* (Cardiologists generally don't treat high LDL-cholesterol or high blood pressure, but there are always exceptions, as DeLinda's story shows.)
- *What are the potential side effects of the medications you're prescribing?* How should I take the drugs? With food? Between meals? At a certain time of day? What should I do if I miss a dose or run out of pills and have forgotten to refill my prescription?
- *When can I expect to see results with my new treatment?* If I am compliant with the medications and I exercise more, lose weight, and eat better, what degree of improvement can I expect?
- *What symptoms should prompt me to see you again before the next scheduled appointment?* (You should also bring up any symptoms you have been having that are out of the ordinary. Maybe you're getting winded more easily doing household chores like changing the sheets or carrying a bag of groceries. Doctors can work with specifics like these to get to a diagnosis—and appropriate treatment—faster.)
- *Is there anyone else in your office I can communicate with if I have questions and you're not available?* A nurse practitioner? A medical partner?
- *Is it best to reach you directly by leaving a message with your receptionist or by e-mailing you?*

Good doctors who will answer your questions, and re-answer them if you don't understand their explanations the first time around, come in both sexes and all ages. What's central is their attitude toward *you*. If you're not comfortable with your doctor or feel she or he gives you short shrift, switch.

HOW YOU TALK TO HEALTH PROFESSIONALS IN THE EMERGENCY ROOM

In the unlikely event that you end up going to the emergency room for heart-related symptoms, there are a number of things you need to know so that you can advocate for yourself most effectively. One is not to delay. We can't stress this enough. If you think, for instance, that there's even a remote chance you are having a heart attack or stroke, don't wait to see whether it passes. And

You May Be More Capable Than You're Told

If you have an unstable condition that puts your health at immediate risk, it's very important to do what your doctor says to get things under control. But if it's a condition that is stable and has been going on for a long time, there's a chance you're more capable of living normally than you may be told.

We have heard a number of stories from people who have gone to see a physician for their hearts and were cautioned not even to break a sweat or lift more than 5 pounds. One active person we know—a jogger and tennis player as well as avid gardener—had a congenital heart murmur that wasn't diagnosed until an annual physical at age 40. Her physician referred her to a cardiologist, who had a cardiology resident examine her via an echocardiogram before coming into the room to follow up. The young resident told her that she was not allowed to lift any weight heavier than 10 pounds and that running was out of the question.

The woman was devastated—her whole life was going to be turned upside down. Fortunately, she brought it up with the cardiologist when he came in to examine her. He told her such advice was unwarranted. She might need a valve replacement many years down the line, he said, but even that was unlikely. If she hadn't spoken up and gotten her "second opinion," she would have walked around on tiptoes—unnecessarily—and suffered a *decline* in her heart health from lack of activity.

don't tell yourself it's nothing. Many women make the dangerous mistake of minimizing what they're going through. This could be a matter of life and death. Delaying can also increase the amount of permanent damage that occurs. *Don't minimize.* Get someone to drive you to the hospital—immediately. If no one's available, call 911.

Once at the hospital, tell the medical team you suspect it's a heart attack or some other heart-related problem. Don't feel funny about it, and don't let anyone tell you it's not possible because you're a woman or because your symptoms are not typical of a heart attack. Remember, women's heart attack symptoms are often diffuse. A heart attack could feel more like indigestion than a train running over your chest. If you have another person with you, so much the better. He or she can fill in where you might not be able to because of pain or anxiety about what's going on.

OUR CHARGE TO YOU

Taking the reins and becoming your own advocate, which in turn makes *others* your advocates, may not be easy. Nor is it easy to change eating and exercise habits that may have been ingrained for decades. But you are at a place in your life where you need to make a decision. You need to weigh whether you are willing to make the necessary changes to improve your heart health, and perhaps even extend your life.

We know you can do it. In the two decades that we have been talking to women about their bodies, we have seen that strong women come in all shapes, ages, sizes, and mind-sets. No matter what their starting point, they have been able to make fundamental shifts in how they live their lives. And the rewards are so worth the effort, as many of the women we spoke with confirmed.

Anne, who was able to take lifestyle steps to lower her cholesterol, says that she could do it because she took charge of her own situation. It was *she* who made sure her doctor finally sent a sample of her blood to a lab for cholesterol analysis. It was also she who got her doctor to pay closer attention to her blood pressure. Because it hadn't quite reached the threshold for "high," her doctor kept telling her not to worry about it. But she kept asking him, "Don't you think it's high for *me,* since I live such a healthy lifestyle?" It was then that closer tabs began to be kept, and they could catch it when it went above 140/90.

Deanne, the woman who improved her heart health by losing weight, says that her best advice "is simply to keep reminding yourself that you can do whatever you want to." A lot of women feel defeated before they even begin, she remarks, but "don't let anyone stand in your way; have confidence in yourself." The payback for that attitude and approach: "I wake up every day and have this incredible feeling of being healthy and happy," Deanne says.

Wendy, who also changed her eating style to keep down her cholesterol, expresses it more bluntly. When you do things right for yourself, she says, "you don't feel 'bad' anymore. You're doing every part of your body, not just your heart, a good favor. The minute I started taking care of my body, I knew that. I know a lot of women think it's hopeless. But it's not. Rant and rave if you have to. Moan about how difficult it is. But then do something about it. You've got to start right now."

We agree. Your life really depends on making the changes. Better still, you will likely enjoy collateral benefits. Women are frequently at the center of their circle of family and friends. How we live our lives often directly impacts how others we care about live theirs. Furthermore, as you make these fundamental changes, you won't feel deprived. Rather, you'll feel enriched because everything you do for yourself you'll be able to do in a way that works within your own lifestyle. The steps are always flexible enough so that you can find a way to adapt them to your needs and tastes.

As you make the shift, which we believe you are doing even by finishing this book, we wish you health and vitality for years to come. We wish you control over your own life. And we wish you a strong heart. From this point forward, it will become stronger still.

Glossary

Aerobic exercise: Continuous exercise that works the entire cardiovascular system, including the heart and lungs, by elevating the heart rate. Examples include brisk walking, running, bicycling, and swimming.

Alpha-linolenic acid (ALA): A type of omega-3 fatty acid found in certain plant foods and plant oils, such as canola and soybean oils, walnuts, and flaxseeds. Only a small amount of ALA can be converted to the type of omega-3s found in fish.

Aneurysm: The abnormal enlargement or bulging of a section of an artery caused by damage to or weakness in the vessel wall. Aneurysms can occur in any type of blood vessel, but they almost always form in an artery.

Angina (an-JI-nuh, or AN-juh-nuh): Chest pain or discomfort that occurs when the heart muscle does not get enough oxygenated blood. It may feel like pressure or a squeezing pain in your chest. The pain may also be felt in the shoulders, arms, neck, jaw, or back. Sometimes it feels like indigestion.

Angioplasty (AN-jee-oh-plas-tee): A medical procedure used to open narrowed or clogged blood vessels of the heart.

Antioxidant: A nutrient or chemical that can "absorb" or block damage caused by substances known as free radicals, thereby protecting body tissue.

Arrhythmia: Refers to any change from the normal sequence of electrical impulses in the heart, causing abnormal heart rhythms.

Arteries: Blood vessels that carry oxygen-rich blood from the heart to all the cells in the body.

Atherosclerosis (ath-er-o-skle-RO-sis): The hardening and narrowing of the arteries caused by the slow buildup of plaque on the inside of the artery walls.

Atrial fibrillation: The heart's two small upper chambers—the left and right atria—quiver instead of beating effectively. Blood isn't pumped completely out of them, so it may pool and clot. If a piece of a blood clot in the atria leaves the heart and becomes lodged in an artery in the brain, a stroke results. About 15 percent of strokes occur in people with atrial fibrillation.

Atrium (right and left) (AY-tree-um): The atria (plural of "atrium") are the two upper chambers of the heart that collect blood as it flows in.

Bicuspid valve: Also known as the mitral (MI-trul) valve, the bicuspid valve is located on the left side of the heart, between the left atrium and the left ventricle.

Blood pressure (systolic and diastolic): The force of the blood pushing against the walls of the arteries as it's pumped out of the heart with each beat. Blood pressure is at its highest when the heart beats, pumping the blood. This is called *systolic pressure*. When the heart is at rest, between beats, your blood pressure falls. This is *diastolic pressure*.

Blood vessels: "Tubes" that carry blood throughout the body. The two main types of blood vessels are arteries and veins. Arteries carry blood *away* from the heart. Veins carry blood back *to* the heart.

Body mass index (BMI): A measure of weight for height. To find your BMI, refer to page 146.

Capillaries: Very small blood vessels that connect arteries to veins. From capillaries, oxygen and nutrients are dropped off by the blood to individual cells. Carbon dioxide and other waste are picked up.

Cardiac catheterization: A catheter, or thin tube, is threaded into the heart, providing information on blood pressure within the heart, how much oxygen is in the blood flowing through the heart, and the pumping ability of the heart.

Cardiovascular system: The entire circulatory system of the body, blood vessels, lungs, and heart.

Carotid artery stenosis (kah-ROT-id AR-ter-ee sten-O-sis): Narrowing of the carotid arteries, the main arteries in the neck that supply blood to the brain. This is a major risk factor for ischemic (is-KEEM-ik) stroke, the most common form of stroke.

Cholesterol: A waxy substance made by the liver and also supplied in the diet through animal foods such as eggs, meats, and dairy products. Cholesterol is needed in the body to insulate nerves, make cell membranes, and produce certain hormones. However, the body can make adequate cholesterol, so dietary cholesterol isn't needed. Dietary cholesterol can raise blood cholesterol, but not nearly as much as saturated fat and *trans*-fatty acids.

Congestive heart failure: A condition wherein the heart cannot efficiently pump blood throughout the body. Excess fluid backs up into the lungs, heart, and other tissues. The fluid collects, causing congestion.

Coronary artery disease (CAD): Occurs when the arteries that supply blood to the heart muscle (coronary arteries) become narrowed or clogged. Blood flow to the heart becomes compromised, decreasing the oxygen supply to the heart muscle.

Daily values: The reference numbers developed by the government that are used for food labeling. The % Daily Value for a nutrient gives a general idea of a food's contribution of that nutrient to the total daily diet.

Docosohexanoic acid (DHA): An omega-3 fatty acid, found in highest concentrations in cold-water fish. Intakes have been related to decreased risk of heart disease.

Eicosapentaenoic acid (EPA): An omega-3 fatty acid, found in highest concentrations in cold-water fish. Intakes have been related to a reduced risk of heart disease.

Fatty acid: A chain of carbons attached to one another with either single or double bonds. A fatty acid with no double bonds is saturated; a chain with a single double bond is monounsaturated; and a chain with two or more double bonds is polyunsaturated. A *trans*-fatty acid contains one or more double bonds in a less common configuration.

Heart attack (myocardial infarction): Occurs when the supply of blood and oxygen to an area of heart muscle is blocked, usually by a clot in a coronary artery. If the blockage is not treated within minutes to hours, the affected heart muscle will die and be replaced by scar. **A heart attack is an emergency. Call 911 if you think you (or someone else) may be having a heart attack. Prompt treatment of a heart attack can help prevent or limit lasting damage to the heart and can also prevent death.**

Heart contractions: Heart muscle squeezing in rhythmic manner to push blood out of the heart. With each contraction, about 50 percent of the blood in the heart is pushed out into the body; less in those with congestive heart failure.

Hemorrhagic stroke: The bursting of an artery in the brain, causing bleeding into the brain.

Inflammation: The process by which the body responds to injury. Laboratory evidence and findings from clinical and population studies suggest that inflammation is part of atherosclerosis, the buildup of fatty deposits in artery linings.

Ischemic stroke: Occurs when a clot blocks blood flow in an artery that brings blood to the brain. Accounts for up to 80 percent of all strokes.

Lipoproteins: These are fat-protein combinations. Because oil (fat) and water (in the blood) don't mix, the fat that circulates in the bloodstream needs to be packaged with protein (and other substances) so it can be transported. The exact makeup of the package determines its role. The three main lipoproteins:

Very Low Density Lipoprotein (VLDL): The major fat-carrying particle in the bloodstream. Delivers fatty acids to all cells in the body for use as energy or storage.

Low Density Lipoprotein (LDL): Commonly referred to as "bad" LDL, it carries most of the cholesterol in the blood, delivering it to cells throughout the body. When LDL delivers excess cholesterol to cells in the walls of blood vessels, atherosclerotic plaque forms.

High Density Lipoprotein (HDL): Commonly referred to as "good" HDL, it's the only lipoprotein particle that carries cholesterol from various cells in the body to the liver for metabolism or excretion.

Mitral valve (See bicuspid valve.)

Murmur: An unusual, or extra, sound heard during your heartbeat. In adults, murmurs are most often due to heart valve problems that cause a little blood to flow backward rather than forward.

Myocardial infarction (See heart attack.)

Omega-3 fatty acids: A family of fatty acids that is essential to human health, found in relatively large quantities in cold-water fish. Also found in certain plant foods and plant oils, such as canola and soybean oils, walnuts, and flaxseeds. Plant-based omega-3s are not as heart-protective. (See also DHA and EPA.)

Peripheral vascular disease: Peripheral vascular disease (PVD) is atherosclerosis of blood vessels other than those of the heart or brain. It predominantly involves the vasculature of the legs or arms. The most common and important type of PVD is peripheral arterial disease, or PAD, which affects 8 to 12 million Americans. It becomes more common as one gets older, and by age 70, about 20 percent of the population is affected. Diagnosis is critical, as people with PAD face a six to seven times higher risk of heart attack or stroke.

Plaque: Made up primarily of cholesterol and sometimes calcium, it can build up inside an artery where, in time, it may restrict blood flow.

Stent: A tiny mesh tube. It is inserted during angioplasty to keep open a narrowed artery. Some stents are coated with medication to help prevent the artery from closing again.

Strength training (progressive resistance training): A mode of exercise in which the muscles work against enough resistance to challenge them and thereby increase strength. An example is weight lifting.

Stroke (See hemorrhagic stroke and ischemic stroke.)

Transient ischemic attack (TIA): A "mini-stroke" that produces strokelike symptoms but no lasting damage. TIAs occur when a blood clot temporarily clogs an artery and part of the brain doesn't get the blood it needs. Symptoms occur rapidly and generally last about one minute.

Tricuspid (tri-CUSS-pid) valve: On the right side of the heart, located between the right atrium and the right ventricle.

Triglycerides: The form of fat found in foods and body fat cells. Triglycerides are used for energy or storage.

Veins: Blood vessels that carry blood back to the heart after it has dropped off oxygen and nutrients throughout the body and picked up waste material, including carbon dioxide.

Ventricles (VEN-trih-kuls): The two lower chambers of the heart that pump blood out of the heart to the lungs or other parts of the body.

Weight-bearing exercise: Aerobic exercises that require the legs to support the weight of the body. Walking is weight-bearing. Swimming and biking are not.

Resources

◆

We list here numerous resources for more information about heart health and related issues. The list includes organizations, books, websites, and more. Please bear in mind that websites frequently change. The sites listed here were accessible when we compiled this section. If any one of them is inoperative at a later date, we encourage you to use a reliable search engine to locate the source at its new site.

General Heart Health Resources

The National Heart, Lung, and Blood Institute (NHLBI) of the National Institutes of Health has a number of excellent websites regarding heart disease. The main website is: www.nhlbi.nih.gov

Specific NHLBI websites are as follows:

The Heart Truth: A National Awareness Campaign for Women About Heart Disease. This is a website sponsored by the U.S. government containing information on heart disease risk specifically in women. www.nhlbi.nih.gov/health/hearttruth

A–Z index on issues related to heart health: www.nhlbi.nih.gov/health/dci Details and suggestions for following the Dietary Approaches to Stop Hypertension (DASH diet): www.nhlbi.nih.gov/health/public/heart/hbp/dash

The American Heart Association (AHA) has an excellent website with information targeted toward consumers. The primary AHA website is: www. americanheart.org

Go to the main AHA website and type in "Go Red for Women" in the search box. This specific website sponsored by the AHA contains information on heart disease risk for women.

Go to the main AHA website and type in "Choose to Move" or "Simple Solutions." These are step-by-step programs to help you become more physically active and choose and prepare heart-healthy foods.

This AHA website provides extensive tips on shopping, cooking, recipes, and general heart-healthy eating: www.deliciousdecisions.org/

The Heart and Stroke Foundation of Canada has an excellent site that contains useful information on heart disease and stroke: ww2.heartandstroke.ca

WomenHeart is an excellent health information and advocacy foundation focused on women and heart disease: www.womenheart.org

Books on Heart Disease and Related Topics

A wide selection of American Heart Association cookbooks is available, ranging from standard heart-healthy recipes to quick and easy meals, meals in minutes, low-fat and low-cholesterol, low-salt, an around-the-world cookbook, and a kid's cookbook. One of them is *To Your Health! A Guide to Heart-Smart Living*, American Heart Association, Random House, 2001.

Women Are Not Small Men: Life-Saving Strategies for Preventing and Healing Heart Disease in Women, Neica Goldberg, M.D., Ballantine Books, 2002.

The Female Heart: The Truth About Women and Heart Disease, Marianne Legato, M.D., and Carol Colman, Perennial Currents, 2000.

Dr. Susan Love's Menopause and Hormone Book: Making Informed Choices, Susan M. Love, M.D., and Karen Lindsay, Three Rivers Press, 2003.

Smoking Cessation

The Department of Health and Human Services provides extensive material on smoking cessation: www.surgeongeneral.gov/tobacco/

Dr. Nelson's Website and Books

www.strongwomen.com has a free electronic newsletter and animated exercise programs as well as other useful information regarding nutrition and exercise.

Strong Women Stay Young (Revised Edition), Miriam E. Nelson, Ph.D., with Sarah Wernick, Ph.D., Bantam Books, 2000.

Strong Women Stay Slim, Miriam E. Nelson, Ph.D., with Sarah Wernick, Ph.D., Bantam Books, 1998.

Strong Women, Strong Bones, Miriam E. Nelson, Ph.D., with Sarah Wernick, Ph.D., Putnam, 2000.

Strong Women Eat Well, Miriam E. Nelson, Ph.D., with Judy Knipe, Putnam, 2001.

Strong Women and Men *Beat Arthritis,* Miriam E. Nelson, Ph.D., Kristin Baker, Ph.D., and Ronenn Roubenoff, M.D., M.S.H., with Lawrence Lindner, M.A., Putnam, 2002.

The Strong Women's Journal, Miriam E. Nelson, Ph.D., Perigee, 2003.

Tufts University Resources

The John Hancock Center for Physical Activity and Nutrition at the Friedman School of Nutrition Science and Policy, Tufts University, maintains a website with useful information regarding ongoing programs such as the community-based StrongWomen Program: www.go.tufts.edu/JHCPAN

In addition, The President's Marathon Challenge at Tufts coordinates and trains runners for the Boston Marathon as part of a large effort to raise awareness and funds for research and outreach on nutrition and physical activity. If you have any interest in joining our team, go to: www.marathon.president.tufts.edu

The Tufts University Health & Nutrition Letter, an eight-page monthly newsletter, has been called "the best available source of news and views on nutrition" by *U.S. News & World Report* and has also received accolades from *The New York Times, The Boston Globe,* and the *Columbia Journalism Review,* among other publications. Go to: www.healthletter.tufts.edu, or call 800-271-7584.

Organizations

The Centers for Disease Control and Prevention provide comprehensive information about nutrition, physical activity, and numerous other health-related topics.

National Center for Chronic Disease Prevention and Health Promotion (NCCDPHP); Division of Nutrition and Physical Activity (DNPA)
  4770 Buford Highway, NE
  Atlanta, GA 30341-3717
  www.cdc.gov/nccdphp/dnpa

The American Dietetic Association lists registered dietitians and provides nutrition information on its website.
  American Dietetic Association
  216 W. Jackson Boulevard
  Chicago, IL 60606-6995
  Ph: 800-366-1655
  www.eatright.org

The National Weight Control Registry has identified more than 4,000 individuals who have lost significant amounts of weight and kept it off for long periods of time: www.lifespan.org/services/bmed/wt_loss/nwcr/

LLuminari is a team of the country's leading health experts. They are highly regarded for their approach to evidence based medicine and their ability to educate, inspire, and energize women to live healthier lives, in body, mind, and spirit. Dr. Nelson is a founding member of the LLuminari Expert Network: www.lluminari.com

The National Strength and Conditioning Association lists certified personal trainers on its website.

National Strength and Conditioning Association
1955 N. Union Boulevard
Colorado Springs, CO 80909
Ph: 719-632-6722 or 800-805-6826
Fax: 719-632-6367
www.nsca.com

The American Council on Exercise is a fitness organization that helps you locate certified exercise professionals in your area.

4851 Paramount Drive
San Diego, CA 92123
800-825-3636
www.acefitness.org

The American College of Sports Medicine conducts research in the field of exercise science and certifies fitness professionals.

P.O. Box 1440
Indianapolis, IN 46206
www.acsm.org

Fifty-Plus Lifelong Fitness is a national organization whose sole mission is the promotion of physical activity for older adults.

P.O. Box 20230
Stanford, CA 94309
650-323-6160
www.50plus.org

America On the Move is a national initiative dedicated to helping individuals and communities across the nation make positive changes to improve health and quality of life.

www.americaonthemove.org.

Shape-Up America! has comprehensive information about nutrition, physical activity, and numerous other health-related topics.

6707 Democracy Boulevard, Suite 306
Bethesda, MD 20817
(301) 493-5368
www.shapeup.org

Books and Other Resources with Reliable Nutrition, Exercise, and Weight Control Information

The American Dietetic Association's Complete Food & Nutrition Guide, Roberta Larson Duyff, M.S., R.D., Chronimed Publishing, 1998.

The Step Diet Book, James Hill, Ph.D., John Peters, Ph.D., with Bonnie Jortberg, M.S., R.D., Workman Publishing, 2004.

The Complete Guide to Walking for Health, Weight Loss, and Fitness, Mark Fenton, The Lyons Press, 2001.

The Spark: A Revolutionary New Plan to Get Fit and Lose Weight, Glenn A. Gaesser, Ph.D., and Karla Dougherty, Simon & Schuster, 2001.

Thin for Life: 10 Keys to Success from People Who Have Lost Weight and Kept It Off, Anne Fletcher, M.S., R.D., Houghton Mifflin Company, 2003.

Stretching 20th Anniversary: An Extensive Book on Stretching, Bob Anderson, Shelten Publishing, August 2000.

Yoga Journal
    Yoga Teachers Directory and Source
    2054 University Avenue
    Berkeley, CA 94704
    Ph: 510-841-9200
    Fax: 510-644-3101
    www.yogajournal.com

Tai Chi Productions
    P.O. Box 752
    Butler, NJ 07405
    Ph: 973-282-9698
    Fax: 800-889-2082
    www.taichiproductions.com

Exercise Equipment

Country Technology, Inc.
    P.O. Box 87
    Gays Mills, WI 54631
    Ph: 608-735-4718
    Fax: 608-735-4859

MC Sports
    3070 Shaffer Street, SE
    Grand Rapids, MI 49512
    Ph: 800-626-1762
    Fax: 616-942-1973

Paragon Sports, Inc.
    867 Broadway
    New York, NY 10003
    Ph: 212-255-8036
    Fax: 212-929-1831

Fitness Distributors
    25 Washington Street
    Natick, MA 01760
    Ph: 800-244-1882 or 508-653-1882
    Fax: 508-650-0448

Australian Barbell Company
   52-54 Bond Street West
   Mordialloc, Victoria, 3195 7123
   Australia
   www.australianbarbellco.com
   E-mail: info@australianbarbellco.com

Digiwalker (reliable pedometer)
   Ph: 888-748-5377
   www.digiwalker.com
   E-mail: info@digiwalker.com

Bibliography

General Heart Disease

Chobanian, A. V., Bakris, G. L., Black, H. R., Cushman, W. C., et al. National High Blood Pressure Education Program Coordinating Committee. Seventh Report of the Joint National Committee on Prevention, Detection, Evaluation, and Treatment of High Blood Pressure. *Hypertension.* 2003; 42: 1206–52.

Expert Panel on Detection, Evaluation, and Treatment of High Blood Cholesterol in Adults. Executive summary of the Third Report of the National Cholesterol Education Program (NCEP) Expert Panel on Detection, Evaluation, and Treatment of High Blood Cholesterol in Adults (Adult Treatment Panel III). *Journal of the American Medical Association.* 2001; 285: 2486–97.

Grundy, S. M., Cleeman, J. I., Merz, C.N., Brewer, B., et al., for the Coordinating Committee of the National Cholesterol Education Program. Implications of Recent Clinical Trials for the National Cholesterol Education Program. Adult Treatment Panel III Guidelines. *Circulation.* 2004; 110: 227–39.

Krauss, R. M., Eckel, R. H., Howard, B., Appel, L. J., et al. American Heart Association Dietary Guidelines: revision 2000: A Statement for Healthcare Professionals from the Nutrition Committee of the American Heart Association. *Circulation* 2002; 102: 2284–99.

Pearson, T. A., Mensah, G. A., Alexander, R. W., Anderson, J. L., et al. Markers of Inflammation and Cardiovascular Disease: Application to Clinical and Public Health Practice: A Statement for Healthcare Professionals from the Centers for Disease Control and Prevention and the American Heart Association. *Circulation.* 2003; 107: 499–511.

Writing Group for the Women's Health Initiative Investigators. Risks and benefits of estrogen plus progestin in healthy postmenopausal women: Principal results from the Women's Health Initiative randomized controlled trial. *JAMA.* 2002; 288: 321–33.

Women and Heart Disease

Angus, J. The material and social predicaments of home: women's experiences after aortocoronary bypass surgery. *Canadian Journal of Nursing Research.* 2001; 33: 27–42.

Lemolo, F., Martiniuk, A., Steinman, D. A., and Spence, J. D. Sex differences in carotid plaque and stenosis. *Stroke.* 2004; 35: 477–81.

Malacrida, R., Genoni, M. Maggioni, A. P., Spataro, V., et al. A comparison of the early outcome of acute myocardial infarction in women and men. The Third International Study of Infarct Survival Collaborative Group. *New England Journal of Medicine.* 1998; 338: 8–14.

McSweeney, J. C., Cody, M., O'Sullivan, P., Elberson, K., et al. Women's early warning symptoms of acute myocardial infarction. *Circulation.* 2003; 108: 2619–23.

Mosca, L., Appel, L. J., Benjamin, E. J., Berra, K., et al. Evidence-based guidelines for cardiovascular disease prevention in women. *Journal of the American College of Cardiology.* 2004; 43: 900–21.

Natarajan, S., Liao, Y., Cao, G., Lipsitz, S. R., and McGee, D. L. Sex differences in risk for coronary heart disease mortality associated with diabetes and established coronary heart disease. *Archives of Internal Medicine.* 2003; 163: 1735–40.

Schulman, K. A., Berlin, J. A., Harless, W., Kerner, J. F., et al. The effect of race and sex on physicians' recommendations for cardiac catheterization. *New England Journal of Medicine.* 1999; 340: 618–26.

Vaccarino, V., Lin, Z. Q., Kasl, S. V., Mattera, J. A., et al. Sex differences in health status after coronary artery bypass surgery. *Circulation* 2003; 108: 2642–47.

Wenger, N. K., Speroff, L., and Packard, B. Cardiovascular health and disease in women. *New England Journal of Medicine.* 1993; 329: 247–56.

Nutrition and Heart Disease

Appel, L. J., Moore, T. J., Obarzanek, E., Vollmer, W. M., et al. A clinical trial of the effects of dietary patterns on blood pressure. *New England Journal of Medicine.* 1997; 336: 1117–24.

Beveridge, J. M. R., Connell, W. F., Mayer, G. A., and Haust, H. L. Plant sterols, degree of unsaturation and hypocholesterolemic action of certain fats. *Canadian Journal of Biochemistry and Physiology.* 1958; 36: 895–911.

Erkkilä, A. T., Lichtenstein, A. H., Mazaffarian, D., and Herrington, D. M. Fish intake is associated with a reduced progression of coronary-artery atherosclerosis in diabetic women with coronary disease. *American Journal of Clinical Nutrition.* 2004; 80: 626–32.

Hu, F. B., Bronner, L., Willett, W. C., Stampfer, M. J., et al. Fish and omega-3 fatty acid intake and risk of coronary heart disease in women. *Journal of the American Medical Association.* 2002; 287: 1815–21.

Jacobs, D. R., Jr., Meyer, K. A., Kushi, L. H., and Folsom, A. R. Whole-grain intake may reduce the risk of ischemic heart disease death in post-menopausal women: the Iowa Women's Health Study. *American Journal of Clinical Nutrition.* 1998; 68: 248–57.

Joshipura, K. J., Hu, F. B., Manson, J. E., Stampfer, M. J., et al. The effect of fruit and vegetable intake on risk for coronary heart disease. *Annals of Internal Medicine.* 2001; 134: 1106–14.

Kushi, L. H., Sc.D., Folsom, A. R., M.D., Prineas, R. J., M.B., B.S., Mink, P. J., M.P.H., et al. Dietary antioxidant vitamins and death from coronary heart disease in postmenopausal women. *New England Journal of Medicine.* 1996; 334: 1156–62.

Lichtenstein, A. H., Ausman, L. M., Carrasco, W., Jenner, J. L., et al. Short-term consumption of a low-fat diet beneficially affects plasma lipid concentrations only when accompanied by weight loss. Hypercholes-terolemia, low-fat diet, and plasma lipids. *Arteriosclerosis & Thrombosis.* 1994; 14: 1751–60.

Lichtenstein, A. H., Ausman, L. A., Jalbert, S. M., and Schaefer, E. J. Comparison of different forms of hydrogenated fats on serum lipid levels in moderately hypercholesterolemic female and male subjects. *New England Journal of Medicine* 1999; 340: 1933–40.

Lichtenstein, A. H., Ausman, L. M., Jalbert, S. M., Vilella-Bach, M., et al. Efficacy of a therapeutic lifestyle change/Step 2 Diet in moderately hypercholesterolemic middle-aged and elderly female and male subjects. *Journal of Lipid Research.* 2002; 43: 264–73.

Lichtenstein, A. H., Jalbert, S. M., Adlercreutz, H., Goldin, B. R., et al. Lipoprotein response to diets high in soy or animal protein with and without isoflavones in moderately hypercholesterolemic subjects. *Arteriosclerosis, Thrombosis & Vascular Biology.* 2002; 22:1852–58.

Lichtenstein, A. H. Dietary fat and cardiovascular disease risk: quantity or quality? *Journal of Women's Health.* 2003; 12: 109–14.

Sacks, F. M., Svetkey, L. P., Vollmer, W. M., Appel, L. J., et al. Effects on blood pressure of reduced dietary sodium and the Dietary Approaches to Stop Hypertension (DASH) Diet. DASH-Sodium Collaborative Research Group. *New England Journal of Medicine.* 2001; 344: 3–10.

Schaefer, E. J., Lichtenstein, A. H., Lamon-Fava, S., Contois, J. H., et al. Efficacy of National Cholesterol Education Program Step 2 Diet in normolipidemic and hypercholesterolemic middle-aged and elderly men and women. *Arteriosclerosis & Thrombosis.* 1995; 15: 1079–85.

Schaefer, E. J. Lipoproteins, nutrition, and heart disease. *American Journal of Clinical Nutrition.* 2002; 75: 191–212.

Physical Activity and Heart Disease

Gulati, M., Pandey, D. K., Arnsdorf, M. F., Lauderdale, D. S., et al. Exercise capacity and the risk of death in women: the St. James Women Take Heart Project. *Circulation.* 2003; 108: 1554–59.

Mora, S., Redberg, R. F., Cui, Y., Whiteman, M. K., et al. Ability of exercise testing to predict cardiovascular and all-cause death in asymptomatic women: a 20-year follow-up of the lipid research clinics prevalence study. *Journal of the American Medical Association.* 2003; 290: 1600–7.

Blair, S. N., Kampert, J. B., Kohl, H. W., III, Barlow, C. E., et al. Influence of cardiovascular fitness and other precursors on cardiovascular disease and all-cause mortality in men and women. *Journal of the American Medical Association.* 1996; 276: 205–10.

Blair, S. N., Kohl, H. W., 3rd, Paffenbarger, R. S., Jr., Clark, D. G., et al. Physical fitness and all-cause mortality: A prospective study of healthy men and women. *Journal of the American Medical Association.* 1989; 262(17): 2395–401.

Castaneda, C., Layne, J., Munoz-Orians, L., Gordon, P., et al. High-intensity progressive resistance exercise training in Hispanic older adults with type 2 diabetes: a randomized controlled trial. *Diabetes Care.* 2002; 25: 2335–41.

Farrell, S. W., Braun, L., Barlow, C. E., Cheng, Y. J., Blair, S. N. The relation of body mass index, cardiorespiratory fitness, and all-cause mortality in women. *Obesity Research.* 2002; 10(6): 417–23.

FitzGerald, S. J., Barlow, C. E., Kampert, J. B., Morrow, J. R., Jr., et al. Muscular fitness and all-cause mortality: prospective observations. *Journal of Physical Activity and Health.* 2004; 1: 7–18.

Hu, F. B., Stampfer, M. J., Colditz, G. A., Ascherio, A., et al. Physical activity and risk of stroke in women. *Journal of the American Medical Association.* 2000; 283(22): 2961–67.

Hu, F. B., Sigal, R. J., Rich-Edwards, J. W., Colditz, G. A., et al. Walking compared with vigorous physical activity and risk of type 2 diabetes in women: a prospective study. *Journal of the American Medical Association.* 1999; 282(15): 1433–39.

Kushi, L. H., Fee, R. M., Folsom, A. R., Mink, P. J., et al. Physical activity and mortality in postmenopausal women. *Journal of the American Medical Association.* 1997; 277(16): 1287–92.

Morris, J. N., Heady, J. A., Raffle, P. A. B., Roberts, C. G., and Parks, J. W. Coronary heart disease and physical activity of work. *The Lancet.* 1953; ii:1053–57.

Paffenbarger, R. S., Jr. Ability of exercise testing to predict cardiovascular and all-cause death in asymptomatic women: a 20-year follow-up of the lipid research clinic's prevalence study. *Journal of the American Medical Association.* 2003; 290: 1600–7.

Paffenbarger, R. S., Jr., Wing, A. L., and Hyde, R. T. Physical activity as an index of heart attack risk in college alumni. *American Journal of Epidemiology.* 1978; 108(3): 161–75.

Tanasescu M., Leitzmann M. F., Rimm, E. B., Willett, W. C., et al. Exercise type and intensity in relation to coronary heart disease in men. *Journal of the American Medical Association.* 2002; 288(16): 1994–2000.

Thompson, P. D., Buchner, D, et al. Exercise and physical activity in the pre-
vention and treatment of atherosclerotic cardiovascular disease: a state-
ment from the Council on Clinical Cardiology (Subcommittee on
Exercise, Rehabilitation, and Prevention) and the Council on Nutrition,
Physical Activity, and Metabolism (Subcommittee on Physical Activity).
Circulation. 2003; 107(24): 3109–16.

Complementary Therapies and Heart Disease
Castillo-Richmond, A., Schneider, R. H., Alexander, C. N., Cook, R., et al.
Effects of stress reduction on carotid atherosclerosis in hypertensive African
Americans. *Stroke.* 2000; 31(3): 568–73.
King, M. S., Carr, T., and D'Cruz, C. Transcendental Meditation, hyper-
tension and heart disease. *Australian Family Physicians.* 2002; 31(2):
164–68.
Liu, E. H., Turner, L. M., Lin, S. X., Klaus, L., et al. Use of alternative medicine
by patients undergoing cardiac surgery. *Journal of Thoracic and Cardiovascular Surgery.* 2000; 120(2): 335–41.
Spigelski, D. B., and Jones, P. J. H. Efficacy of garlic supplementation in lowering serum cholesterol levels. *Nutrition Reviews.* 2001; 59(7): 236–41.
Zamarra, J. W., Schneider, R. H., Besseghini, I., Robinson, D. K., and Salerno,
J. W. Usefulness of the Transcendental Meditation program in the treatment of patients with coronary artery disease. *American Journal of Cardiology.* 1996; 77(10): 867–70.

Acknowledgments

---◆---

The names you see on a book cover represent but a small fraction of the people involved in bringing a work to fruition.

We first express our gratitude to Lawrence Bacow, president of Tufts University, for his leadership in bringing nutrition and physical activity to the forefront of the university's mission—and for providing the best example, through his participation in the annual President's Marathon Challenge, of how even the busiest people can find time to take care of themselves through training and eating well.

A number of other present as well as past colleagues at Tufts, many of whom double as close friends, have also buoyed our efforts along the way. Heartfelt appreciation goes to Drs. Eileen Kennedy, Irwin Rosenberg, Christina Economos, Jeanne Goldberg, Aviva Must, Raymond Hyatt, Roger Fielding, Ronenn Roubenoff, Carmen Castenada Sceppa, Kristin Baker, Lynne Ausman, Sarah Booth, Arja Erkkila, Nirupa Matthan, Simin Meydan, Ursula Schwab, Susan Roberts, and Sonia Vega Lopez. The entire good-hearted staff who work with Miriam at Tufts's John Hancock Center for Physical Activity and Nutrition and with Alice at the Cardiovascular Nutrition Laboratory at the Jean Mayer USDA Human Nutrition Research Center on Aging at Tufts have our sincere gratitude.

A special thanks from Alice to Ernst Schaefer, M.D., for the mentoring along with all the encouragement and opportunities he has provided. Also, thanks that can't be adequately expressed in words go to D. Mark Hegsted,

Ph.D., doctoral thesis adviser to Alice, who has served as a scientific moral role model all these years.

Susan Jalbert must also be mentioned here for single-handedly dealing with all the day-to-day issues of running the Cardiovascular Nutrition Laboratory. There is nothing she wouldn't do to get the job done right. Rebecca Seguin deserves special recognition. She provided invaluable assistance analyzing numerous menus to help us get just right the nutrition program in this book. We express gratitude as well to Nilda Martin and Lori Ioannone, who ably helped with administrative details. Appreciation also goes to Franci Otting, who served as a model for some of the exercise illustrations.

Many thanks to colleague Daniel Forman, M.D., a cardiologist at Harvard Medical School, who graciously agreed to vet this book for us, providing top-notch help with accuracy and details. Any errors that might remain are ours alone.

Of course, without our colleagues at Putnam, none of this could have happened. We salute our editor, Marian Lizzi, for her keen eye and guidance throughout the editing process. And much appreciation goes to all the able individuals in Putnam's publicity department who do their utmost—and always have—to make sure *Strong Women* stays in the news.

Of Wendy Weil, our friend and warmhearted agent, we cannot come up with enough superlatives to thank her for her support through all seven *Strong Women* books. As always, we thank Wendy Wray for her incredible illustrations.

We are indebted to those who fund our research. There are many, but we want to recognize in particular here the National Institutes of Health, the U.S. Department of Agriculture, John Hancock Financial Services, Inc., and the New Balance Foundation.

Individual thanks go from Miriam to Gary Hirshberg at Stonyfield Farms for his help to further the *Strong Women* movement. In addition, Neill Walsdorf, Jr., and his colleagues at Mission Pharmacal have greatly enhanced the visibility of *Strong Women* worldwide.

Collaborator Larry Lindner's writing colleagues Gail Zyla, Anne Fletcher, Christine Smith, and Mary Thang will never know how important they have been and continue to be. Especially grateful thanks go to Joanna Standley, a young friend with an old soul.

To the people who agreed to be interviewed for this book, thank you for your help in putting voices to the drama of heart disease. Linda, Wendy, Deanne, DeLinda, Kim, Cindy, Helen, Pearl, Judy, and Anne have contributed greatly through their candor and patience. So has Nancy Loving, executive director of WomenHeart, who helped put us in touch with some of the women we spoke to.

Larry wishes to thank Shirley Lindner, whose heart is at the heart of everything good; Rochelle and Patricia Lindner, who have been instrumental in bringing joy to our family of men; and the next generation of Lindner women: Kimberly, Heidi, Melanie, Sarah, and Amanda. Weren't you all girls just five minutes ago?

As for our spouses, "thanks" is hardly the word. To Kin Earle, for *always* providing Miriam the support and the freedom that lets her pursue this incredible *Strong Women* journey; to Barry Goldin, for his unwavering confidence in Alice's abilities and for encouraging her to go far beyond what she ever envisioned she could do; and to Constance Lindner. Without Constance, there's no Larry.

Finally, while for obvious reasons this book is dedicated to our daughters, Eliza Earle, Alexandra Earle, and Rachel Lichtenstein Goldin, we are equally dedicated to our sons—Mason Earle, David Lichtenstein Goldin, and John Lindner. You guys—firstborns, all of you—are the ones who gave us our initial lessons in just how rich and full a heart can grow.

Index

ABOUT THE AUTHORS

Miriam Nelson, Ph.D., is director of the John Hancock Center for Physical Activity and Nutrition and associate professor of nutrition at the Friedman School of Nutrition Science and Policy, Tufts University. She is also a fellow of the American College of Sports Medicine, an honor reserved for those who have demonstrated leadership and research in the field of exercise.

For the last fifteen years, Dr. Nelson has been the principal investigator of studies on exercise and nutrition, work supported by grants from the government and private foundations. During this time she was named a Brookdale National Fellow, a prestigious award given annually to only five or six young scholars deemed to be future leaders in the field of aging. She was also awarded a Bunting Fellowship at the Mary Ingraham Bunting Institute at Radcliffe College. In 1998, Dr. Nelson received the Lifetime Achievement Award from the Massachusetts Governor's Committee on Physical Fitness and Sports.

Dr. Nelson is the author of the international best sellers *Strong Women Stay Young*; *Strong Women Stay Slim*; *Strong Women, Strong Bones*; *Strong Women Eat Well*; and *Strong Women* and Men *Beat Arthritis*. She also recently released *The Strong Women's Journal*. These titles, published in fourteen languages, have sold more than a million copies worldwide. *Strong Women, Strong Bones* received the esteemed "Books for a Better Life Award" for best wellness book of 2000 from the Multiple Sclerosis Society.

In August 2001, Dr. Nelson appeared in her own PBS special entitled "Strong Women Live Well," which focused on the benefits of exercise and nutrition for women's health. She has been featured on many television and radio shows, including *The Oprah Winfrey Show*, *The Today Show*, *Good Morning America*, ABC Nightly News, CNN, Fresh Air, and the Discovery

Channel. Dr. Nelson is a motivational speaker who lectures about women's health around the world. She is also a LLuminari health expert.

She lives in Concord, Massachusetts, with her husband and three children.

Alice H. Lichtenstein, D.Sc., is the Stanley N. Gershoff Professor of Nutrition Science and Policy in the Friedman School at Tufts University, and director of the Cardiovascular Nutrition Laboratory at the Jean Mayer USDA Human Nutrition Research Center on Aging at Tufts. Dr. Lichtenstein holds a secondary appointment as professor of family medicine and community health at Tufts University School of Medicine. In June 2005 she will receive an honorary doctoral degree from the Faculty of Medicine, University of Kuopio, Finland.

Dr. Lichtenstein has been the principal investigator of numerous National Institutes of Health– and American Heart Association–funded studies addressing the relationship between diet and heart disease risk factors. She has coauthored more than 100 peer-reviewed articles, thirty review articles, and twenty book chapters on nutrition and heart disease and related topics.

Dr. Lichtenstein served on the USDA/HHS 2000 Dietary Guidelines Advisory Committee and the Dietary Reference Intake Macronutrient Panel of the National Academy of Sciences, Institute of Medicine, Food and Nutrition Board. She currently serves as chair, Nutrition Committee, American Heart Association. She is also a fellow of the Nutrition, Physical Activity and Metabolism Council and the Arteriosclerosis, Thrombosis and Vascular Biology Council of the American Heart Association. In addition, she is a member of the American Society of Nutritional Sciences and the American Society of Clinical Nutrition.

She has served on the editorial board of the *Journal of Nutrition* and is currently serving on the editorial board of *Atherosclerosis*; as an associate editor for the *Journal of Lipid Research*; and as a member of the editorial advisory boards of the *Journal of Nutrition in Clinical Care* and the *Tufts University Health & Nutrition Letter*. Dr. Lichtenstein frequently comments on nutrition-related issues in the popular press, including *The New York Times, Washington Post, Newsweek,* and *Time* magazine. She has also appeared on numerous national television shows, including *The Today Show* and CNN news.

She lives in Newton, Massachusetts, with her husband and two children.

Lawrence Lindner, M.A., writes a regular column for the *Boston Globe.* He also penned the "Eating Right" column for the *Washington Post* for several years and currently freelances for a variety of magazines on health, travel, and other subjects. He lives in Hingham, Massachusetts, with his wife and son.

To contact Dr. Nelson, please send letters to:
Miriam E. Nelson, Ph.D.
Director, John Hancock Center for Physical Activity and Nutrition
Friedman School of Nutrition Science and Policy
Tufts University
150 Harrison Avenue
Boston, MA 02111

Dr. Nelson regrets that, due to the volume of mail she receives, she cannot respond personally to every letter.

Please visit: www.strongwomen.com